THE
EVERYTHING®
GUIDE TO
GLP-1s

Lose Weight, Build Healthy Eating Habits, and Achieve Lifelong Weight Management

KAYLEY GEORGE, MS, RDN

Adams Media

New York   Amsterdam/Antwerp   London   Toronto   Sydney/Melbourne   New Delhi

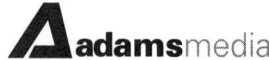

Adams Media
An Imprint of Simon & Schuster, LLC
100 Technology Center Drive
Stoughton, MA 02072

For information about special discounts for bulk purchases, please contact Simon & Schuster Special Sales at 1-866-506-1949 or business@simonandschuster.com.

The Simon & Schuster Speakers Bureau can bring authors to your live event. For more information or to book an event, contact the Simon & Schuster Speakers Bureau at 1-866-248-3049 or visit our website at www.simonspeakers.com.

Interior layout by Maya Caspi and Colleen Cunningham
Nutritional analysis by Mitali Shah-Bixby

Manufactured in the United States of America

1 2025

Library of Congress Cataloging-in-Publication Data
Names: George, Kayley, author.
Title: The everything® guide to GLP-1s / Kayley George, MS, RDN.
Description: First Adams Media trade paperback edition. | Stoughton, Massachusetts: Adams Media, 2025. | Series: Everything® series | Includes bibliographical references and index.
Identifiers: LCCN 2024057532 | ISBN 9781507223833 (pb) | ISBN 9781507223840 (ebook)
Subjects: LCSH: Weight loss. | Reducing diets. | Glucagon-like peptide 1--Agonists--Therapeutic use. | Appetite depressants. | Semaglutide.
Classification: LCC RM222.2 .G4457 2025 | DDC 613.2/5--dc23/eng/20250118
LC record available at https://lccn.loc.gov/2024057532

ISBN 978-1-5072-2383-3
ISBN 978-1-5072-2384-0 (ebook)

Dear Reader,

Whether you're just beginning your GLP-1 journey or looking for additional support along the way, you've come to the right place! *The Everything® Guide to GLP-1s* was created to help you navigate this exciting new class of weight loss medications with confidence.

If you're one of the millions who have taken the significant step of starting GLP-1s yet feel unsure about managing your eating habits, coping with symptoms, building a healthy lifestyle, and keeping the weight off, know that you're not alone. Many people start on GLP-1s without the necessary resources or guidance to make it a **lasting success**—and too often, the excess weight returns. Without support, the "miracle" drug can provide only short-term success, and it can feel like yet another failed diet plan. But it doesn't have to be that way.

I wrote this book to empower and equip you with the essential knowledge and tools that are often overlooked. I'll guide you toward becoming one of the 33 percent who **successfully maintain** their weight loss after using these medications. As a registered dietitian with a passion for healthy, sustainable weight management, I believe that true, lasting weight loss doesn't require restrictive diets or drastic measures—and that you don't need to sacrifice your mental health for the sake of your **physical health**, either. When paired with effective diet and lifestyle changes, this new class of GLP-1 medications can truly be transformative.

Together, let's work toward a lasting success story. Are you ready to join me?

Kayley George, MS, RDN

Welcome to the Everything® Series!

These handy, accessible books give you all you need to tackle a difficult project, gain a new hobby, comprehend a fascinating topic, prepare for an exam, or even brush up on something you learned back in school but have since forgotten.

You can choose to read an Everything® book from cover to cover or just pick out the information you want from our four useful boxes: Questions, Facts, Alerts, and Essentials. We give you everything you need to know on the subject, but throw in a lot of fun stuff along the way too.

QUESTION
Answers to common questions.

FACT
Important snippets of information.

ALERT
Urgent warnings.

ESSENTIAL
Quick handy tips.

We now have more than 600 Everything® books in print, spanning such wide-ranging categories as cooking, health, parenting, personal finance, wedding planning, word puzzles, and so much more. When you're done reading them all, you can finally say you know Everything®!

PUBLISHER Karen Cooper

ASSOCIATE COPY DIRECTOR Casey Ebert

PRODUCTION EDITOR Jo-Anne Duhamel

SENIOR CONTENT EDITOR Lisa Laing

EVERYTHING® SERIES COVER DESIGNER Erin Alexander

Dedication

A special thank-you to my mom, the
true author of this family, for your guidance
throughout this book and my life. To my dad, for your
endless support, and to my sister, for always
bringing love and laughter.

Contents

CHAPTER 9

Snacks 175

CHAPTER 10

Dessert 191

Acknowledgments

Writing this book has been an unexpected and incredible journey, and it would not have been possible without the support of so many remarkable people.

First, to my mom, the true author of this family—your unwavering belief in me and your guidance throughout my life and this process has been my greatest gift.

To Ryan, thank you for holding everything together, always taking care of me, and pushing me across the finish line. You are my rock!

To my friends, thank you for your constant encouragement. You've always been my biggest cheerleaders.

To my team, thank you for giving me the space and support to take on this project. Your dedication to our clients during this time has been invaluable, and I couldn't have done it without you all.

A heartfelt thank you to Julia, Lisa, and the entire publishing team. Your expertise, meticulous attention to detail, and gracious support have been instrumental in shaping this book into what it is today. I am deeply grateful for this opportunity.

And to all the readers—thank you for picking up this book. I hope it resonates with you and helps guide you to become the best version of yourself.

With deepest gratitude,
Kayley

Introduction

Welcome to the new era of weight loss medications. In recent years, a ground-breaking class of glucagon-like peptide-1 (GLP-1) receptor agonist drugs have revolutionized the weight loss industry, exceeding all expectations—both medically and financially. These drugs mimic a peptide created naturally in the small intestine that can lower blood sugar and enhance insulin secretion. When it became clear that the medication resulted in substantial weight loss, what began as a new approach to treating type 2 diabetes turned into a $100 billion industry, reshaping how we approach weight loss.

Weight loss is no longer viewed solely as a battle of sheer willpower and strict dietary restrictions. The oversimplified mantra of "eat less, exercise more" is being replaced by a nuanced understanding of metabolism and human psychology. The era of viewing weight loss through a simple in-and-out caloric formula is fading, making way for a more comprehensive approach.

As research evolves, it's becoming apparent that weight loss requires a multifaceted behavioral, physical, and psychological approach. Weight loss should be tailored to the individual, rather than relying on an arbitrary set of rules about what you can and cannot eat. The weight loss industry was ripe for a new solution. In June 2021, the FDA's approval of semaglutide (marketed as Wegovy) marked a pivotal moment, heralding a new chapter in weight loss treatment. GLP-1 mimicking drugs like semaglutide have emerged as game changers, aligning with natural metabolic functions and targeting multiple facets of weight loss at once.

This book explores how the GLP-1 hormone has emerged as the stand-out solution for weight loss, surpassing other hormones and previous drug iterations. You'll discover how to optimize the results of your medications with a diet and lifestyle plan specifically designed for GLP-1s—a completely different approach from any weight loss attempts you've tried before. In Chapters 2 and 3, read about how to calculate your nutritional needs, which foods to eat (and which ones to avoid), and how to create lasting healthy habits. You'll also be prepared for weaning off the medication and keeping the weight off in the long term.

While it's easy to talk about what you should eat, it's another thing to make it a reality. To keep you on track during your weight loss journey, this book includes 125 delicious dietitian-curated recipes to try out. No more scrolling through Pinterest or going down the Google rabbit hole trying to figure out what to cook—everything you need is right here. These easy-to-make recipes include a balanced variety of ingredients: lean protein for maintaining muscle mass, fresh vegetables and fruits to add essential nutrients and keep you hydrated, and fiber-rich whole grains for healthy digestion. Try make-ahead "Sausage" Egg Cups or an easy (and stomach-soothing) Cinnamon Smoothie. Simple, flavorful meals, like Ginger Chicken Salad and Pineapple Shrimp Fried Rice, will tempt your appetite. And you'll even find recipes for small snacks and desserts, including Fruit and Cheese Kebabs and Pumpkin Blondies. As a bonus, you'll find six GLP-1 specific meal plans that offer practical examples of how to eat throughout the week.

By choosing this book, you're already on the right track to a healthy, sustainable weight loss journey. It's a step toward prioritizing your health and well-being in a time when it's all too easy to lose yourself while caring for others and managing everything else in life. There will be good days and bad days, but don't forget the reasons that inspired you to begin this journey in the first place. You've got this! Let's get started learning about how GLP-1 medications can help you to take charge of your own health, lose weight, and keep it off.

CHAPTER 1

An Introduction to GLP-1s

Obesity is an ever-growing public health crisis, affecting millions and contributing to several life-threatening conditions such as diabetes, heart disease, and even cancer. Despite countless diets, treatments, and medications that have been developed to address it, the prevalence of obesity persists. Traditional methods have failed to provide long-term results for many people, and weight loss drugs developed over the past decades ranged from ineffective to downright dangerous. But recently, the advent of glucagon-like peptide-1 (GLP-1) receptor agonists has generated major excitement in the medical world. Originally developed to treat type 2 diabetes, these medications are showing real promise in reducing cases of obesity. With GLP-1s, losing weight isn't a distant dream—it's a science-supported, achievable reality. These drugs are changing the game for weight and health management, finally providing a solid answer to a problem that has seemed impossible to solve for too long. Now, there's no turning back on this new era of weight loss! Let's take a look at how this wonder drug came to be and how it can help you.

How Did We Get Here?

Obesity is widely accepted as the largest and fastest growing public health concern in the developed world. The condition is considered a contributing factor in over 300,000 annual deaths in the United States alone, according the National Institutes of Health. Data from the 2018 National Health and Nutrition Examination Survey (NHANES) showed that roughly 42 percent of American adults have obesity and about 30 percent are overweight. Combined, that adds up to more than 70 percent of the population. Having excess body weight is not just a problem on its own. It can lead to several other serious health conditions, including cardiovascular disease, cancer, diabetes, kidney disease, arthritis, and gallstones, among other conditions.

To tackle this health pattern, people have been inundated with weight loss diets, medications, and treatments. From the first diet book ever published (*The Art of Living Long* by Luigi Cornaro) in 1558 to the complex bariatric surgeries of today, there has been no shortage of options to try to lose weight. A recent survey conducted by YouGov.com found that at least 60 percent of Americans want to lose weight at some point and half of those are always trying to do so. This overwhelming demand for weight loss has culminated in a $72 billion diet industry that, unfortunately, has not curbed the rising rates of obesity. If anything, it's only caused confusion.

FACT

Early versions of weight loss medications were combination pills that blended several mechanisms, or even several classes of medications, into one drug. Rainbow pills, named for their bright colors, combined amphetamines, diuretics, laxatives, and thyroid hormones to maximize weight loss. Rainbow pills were ultimately removed from the market in the 1960s due to a rising number of adverse effects, such as congestive heart failure and hyperthyroidism, and deaths associated with their use.

For decades, society has presented conflicting theories about weight loss. In the mid-twentieth century, many people attempted a low-fat diet, avoiding butter, cream, and red meat. In 1992, the USDA unveiled its food pyramid, which recommended consuming 6–11 servings of grains daily, but soon after that, keto and Paleo diets gained in popularity. These diets advised avoiding almost all carbohydrates and eating foods that are high in fat. It's no wonder people are always searching for new solutions to cut through the confusion.

Even recent, mainstream approaches to weight loss, such as Weight-Watchers, have left people struggling. A study published in 2023 following WeightWatchers participants found that 43 percent of users gained back 5 or more pounds a year after finishing the program. The two main factors contributing to regaining weight were a lack of sustained high activity levels and the failure to self-monitor food intake (such as through food journaling or point tracking). It appears that most weight loss programs work when you are actively participating in them. Understandably, most people can't keep up with tracking "points" and reporting every bite of food they consume, so these weight loss attempts also prove unsustainable.

FACT

Hormones, primarily ghrelin and leptin, regulate appetite and energy balance. Ghrelin, produced in the stomach, signals hunger to the brain, increasing appetite. Leptin, made by fat cells, signals fullness and reduces appetite. An imbalance between these hormones can disrupt hunger cues, leading to overeating, weight gain, or difficulty maintaining a healthy diet.

Pharmaceutical companies also attempted to provide answers to the diet enigma. However, most of their attempts to solve the riddle were dead ends. Most of their drug options either lacked long-lasting success or had such severe side effects that they had to be shelved. For example, amphetamines were a popular product until medical professionals discovered their addictive tendencies and potential for organ damage.

The 1990s saw the quick rise and fall of fen-phen, a combination of phentermine and fenfluramine. The medication was withdrawn in 1997 after it was linked to severe heart and lung damage. These failed products were revamped into our modern version of appetite suppressants, the most well-known being phentermine. However, even the most refined versions of these suppressants only boast an initial weight loss of 3 percent of body weight among users. Several scientists also experimented with manipulating different hormones, such as leptin (satiety hormone) and ghrelin (hunger hormone), looking for the magic bullet but to no avail.

Historically, obesity has been deemed a behavioral or willpower problem rather than a metabolic disease, so researchers struggled to get funding, which limited their progress. It seemed there wasn't much hope on the horizon until a new class of medications—GLP-1s—entered the picture.

What Are GLP-1s?

Unbeknownst to the public, there was a new pharmaceutical solution in the works that proved to be a larger phenomenon than anyone could have predicted: a new class of medications called glucagon-like peptide-1 (GLP-1) receptor agonists, commonly referred to by the brand names Ozempic or Wegovy. You may see these drugs referred to as GLP-1RAs, but for the purposes of this book, the entire class of GLP-1 receptor agonists will be referred to as "GLP-1s." The discovery of the GLP-1 hormone dates back to the 1980s, when Dr. Joel Habener at Massachusetts General Hospital identified that the proglucagon gene in the small intestine produced not only glucagon (a hormone that raises blood sugar) but also GLP-1, a peptide that can lower blood sugar and enhance insulin secretion in response to food intake. The discovery of GLP-1 opened the door for the development of GLP-1 receptor agonists, medications designed to mimic the hormone's effects.

Dr. Habener found that the first version of injectable GLP-1 was metabolized before it could reach the pancreas. For years, his team tried to find a workaround, but to no avail. It wasn't until a chemist, Dr. Lotte Bjerre Knudsen, at Novo Nordisk successfully attached GLP-1 to a blood protein that it was able to remain in the bloodstream for 24 hours. In 2010, one of the first GLP-1 drugs, liraglutide, was developed for use in controlling blood sugar levels. The medication was a step in the right direction but had disappointing weight loss results, so the Novo Nordisk team went back to the drawing board.

ESSENTIAL

Many researchers worked on GLP-1 research at the same time as Dr. Habener. Dr. Jens Juul Holst was in the same pursuit at the University of Copenhagen, as well as Dr. Daniel Drucker from Mount Sinai Hospital. Each of these scientists has produced integral research on the GLP-1 hormone. Dr. Habener focused on genetics, and Dr. Drucker studied transgenic mice. Dr. Holst concentrated on clinical research related to hormones like insulin and glucagon, discovering the GLP-1 hormone sequence almost simultaneously with Dr. Habener.

In 2017, the breakthrough that researchers had been striving for finally arrived. A high-dose long-lasting injectable, semaglutide (brand name Ozempic), hit the market with remarkable results for patients with type 2 diabetes. The initial SUSTAIN trial in 2017 demonstrated that A1C levels, a key marker used to measure blood sugar, were reduced an average of 20 percent over a three-month period. The weekly injectable also led to a 15 percent weight loss in patients. Physicians and pharmaceutical companies soon realized the broader application of the drug beyond managing diabetes. In June 2021, semaglutide use was expanded by the FDA for long-term weight management in adults with obesity—with the new name of Wegovy.

The response to the medication was nothing short of historic; so much so that a team of analysts at Morgan Stanley predicted 7 percent of the entire population will take the medication over the next ten years. Not only does this medication serve as an effective tool against obesity, but it also offers a range of other positive health outcomes. Research has found that users experience a decrease in hemoglobin A1C (HbA1c), lower fasting glucose levels, enhanced insulin sensitivity, and improved beta cell function—the cells responsible for regulating blood sugar levels. GLP-1 medications are now indicated for reducing the risk of heart attack and cardiovascular disease. Other benefits include improved sleep apnea, better blood pressure, and reduced risk of kidney disease. Remarkably, users have also noted drinking less alcohol and smoking less, likely resulting from the medication working on dopamine pathways.

The medication affects a few different mechanisms in the body, including blood sugar levels and hunger hormones. Many users also believe that the injection turns down the "food noise," the constant preoccupation with food that can lead to mindless eating. With several metabolic pathways better regulated, this medication creates the perfect storm for weight loss with the results to back it up.

Approximately 85 percent of people taking a GLP-1 medication lose at least 5 percent of their starting weight and can expect around 15 percent body weight loss overall—three times the weight loss seen from its predecessor, liraglutide. With these results, GLP-1 medications have become blockbuster drugs, exceeding all expectations and ushering us into a new era of weight loss.

How Do They Work?

The GLP-1 agonists on the market today help regulate blood sugar by acting like the GLP-1 hormone your body naturally produces. These physician-prescribed medications are self-injected weekly under the skin. Typically, patients begin with a low dose, which is gradually increased as their bodies acclimate to the medication. Healthcare providers observe patients to find the sweet spot of dosing that balances effective weight loss and minimal side effects.

FACT

According to Novo Nordisk, semaglutide is almost identical (94 percent) to the natural GLP-1 hormone, which is a small protein made up of 30 building blocks called amino acids. The natural version of this hormone doesn't last long in the body. To develop semaglutide, scientists made small changes to the structure of the hormone to prevent it from being broken down so quickly, slow down its removal by the kidneys, and let it stay in the body longer.

Natural GLP-1 Hormone

One of the main roles of GLP-1 is to regulate your blood sugar, also known as glucose. Keeping blood sugar balanced is foundational for sustainable weight loss. Your blood sugar levels are largely determined by the foods you eat but can also be influenced by other lifestyle choices, such as exercise, sleep, and stress. Blood sugar can also fluctuate based on food timing, menstrual cycles, medications, alcohol, smoking, and caffeine.

Every food has a different impact on blood sugar. This phenomenon has been captured by a model called the glycemic index (GI) that rates foods on their glycemic response as low, medium, or high. Carbohydrate-rich foods, such as grains, fruit, and starchy vegetables, are the primary players that increase blood sugar levels and, subsequently, trigger the release of insulin. In contrast, protein and fat have a minimal effect on blood sugar levels and instead are known for their stabilizing benefits. The GI model will be discussed in more detail in Chapter 2.

The regulation of blood sugar is a complex process in the body, managed by the small intestine, liver, and pancreas, which is where the majority of GLP-1 receptors are found. Your body works day and night to keep everything running in harmony, a state also called homeostasis. The sweet spot for blood sugar is 80–120 mg/dL. When this system is out of balance—with high or low blood sugar levels—it can make it harder to lose weight.

QUESTION

How can the same foods produce different blood sugar responses?

The GI value of any particular food describes the average person's blood sugar response. Individual responses to the same food can vary among different people, and you might even see fluctuating responses after eating the same exact foods. Many factors affect the body's glycemic response. For example, your blood sugar after a meal could look different based on your current stress levels, when you last worked out, how you slept the night before, or where you are in your monthly cycle. Even the other foods you eat along with a carbohydrate can affect the body's response.

Insulin Resistance

When you have excess blood sugar in circulation, your body releases insulin, the hormone that tells your cells to soak up glucose from the blood. That rise in insulin signals the body to slow down on burning fat and instead start storing it. The liver and the muscles take on as much glucose as they can and then turn to fat cells to take on the rest. Fat cells serve as long-term storage for excess glucose, which is converted into chains of fat known as triglycerides and stored until the body experiences an energy shortage. Over time, chronically high blood sugar develops into a condition called insulin resistance. When your body is insulin resistant, it stops responding to incoming blood sugar as it normally would. In response, your body pumps out more and more insulin to override the system, which only makes matters worse. With insulin levels running rampant, weight loss becomes significantly more challenging. Elevated blood sugar also brings along other unwanted symptoms, including a weakened immune system, damage to blood vessels, and problems with the kidneys, eyes, gums, feet, and nerves.

Synthetic GLP

GLP-1 medications contain synthetic GLP-1 hormones that dock on the GLP-1 receptors in the gastrointestinal tract, liver, pancreas, and brain. This analog hormone was developed to stay on the receptor significantly longer than the natural hormone and be more resistant to breakdown. To put this in perspective, the half-life of the natural, or native, GLP-1 is a few minutes, while semaglutide has a half-life of 168 hours, or nearly seven days.

When insulin levels are lower, the body becomes more receptive to burning fat. The GLP-1 hormone keeps the body in this fat-burning state by improving insulin sensitivity, reducing the production of glucose by the liver, and slowing down digestion to promote a feeling of satiety. When food moves through the digestive tract more slowly, your body continues blasting out signals that it's full. Because the drug suppresses your appetite and keeps you feeling fuller for longer, you end up eating less and staying in a caloric deficit (you're burning more calories than you consume).

GLP-1 medication doesn't magically burn fat. It keeps blood sugar balanced and helps to maintain a significant caloric deficit, which is necessary for weight loss.

Outside of working on the digestive tract, GLP-1 also has receptors in different areas of the brain. These brain receptors are likely the reason the drugs can curb the desire to eat. Users have referred to this as turning off the "food noise" or the constant overthinking about what to eat. Research is also emerging showing that GLP-1 may curb addictive tendencies, such as drinking, smoking, taking drugs, or even excess spending. Some experts suggest that GLP-1 is most effective because of its work on the brain.

Other Similar Medications

Tirzepatide is another popular prescription medication that acts in a similar fashion to semaglutide medications. Tirzepatide is marketed under the brand name Mounjaro for individuals with type 2 diabetes and Zepbound for chronic weight management. Semaglutide only works on the GLP-1 hormone, while tirzepatide mimics both the GLP-1 hormone and another hormone, glucose-dependent insulinotropic polypeptide (GIP), which both help regulate blood sugar and appetite. To be specific, GIP helps to increase your insulin sensitivity, while GLP-1 increases your insulin secretion. Basically, you'll be making more insulin and your body will be more receptive to it. Like semaglutide, tirzepatide is prescribed as a weekly injection and available in various dosage strengths.

ALERT

When commercial versions of a drug are difficult to obtain, often due to high demand, compounding pharmacies are allowed to make similar medications to fill the gap. However, these medications are not FDA-approved, and they don't go through the same rigorous safety and efficacy testing as brand-name drugs. And some vendors may use non-FDA-approved ingredients or operate in legal gray areas, putting patients at risk. Consult a healthcare provider before considering a compounded version to ensure you're making a safe and informed decision.

Novo Nordisk and other drug manufacturers are also developing versions of GLP-1 that can be administered orally instead of by injection. As of 2024, the company has a pill version of semaglutide called Rybelsus. Based on clinical trials, Rybelsus is somewhat less effective than its injectable counterpart, Ozempic. However, manufacturers are actively researching more effective tablet versions of GLP-1 to reach more users who are hesitant to use injections.

As of this writing, another iteration of the drug called retatrutide is currently in development, which would mimic a third hormone: glucagon. (In medical circles, this is called a triagonist medication.) While it's still in its early stages of development, the results look promising—an average weight loss of 24 percent of body weight after forty-eight weeks on the medication. It's clear that researchers have only scratched the surface of the possibilities of GLP-1 variations.

Who Can Benefit from GLP-1 Medications?

GLP-1 medications were originally created to help people with type 2 diabetes manage diabetes markers such as A1C, fasting blood sugar, and postprandial blood sugar—the blood sugar level measured after eating. However, as their effectiveness in weight loss became evident, manufacturers expanded their use with higher doses and broader indications. While you and your physician will decide if and which medications are appropriate for you, GLP-1 prescriptions are typically prescribed to individuals with a body mass index (BMI) classified as obese (BMI greater than or equal to 30) or as overweight (BMI greater than or equal to 27), with other weight-related symptoms.

In addition to facilitating weight loss, a lesser-known feature of GLP-1 is its role in curbing chronic inflammation—an ongoing heightened immune system reaction when there is no longer an infection or injury—in the body. Gastroenterologists are exploring its use to treat highly inflammatory conditions like ulcerative colitis and Crohn's disease (in cases where the individual is not underweight). High levels of inflammation hamper the body's ability to process insulin, creating a snowball reaction of rising blood sugar levels and weight. For individuals with high inflammation and a high BMI, GLP-1 can be a great tool to address both.

ALERT

GLP-1s are not appropriate for everyone. They should not be taken during pregnancy. People living with certain conditions, including thyroid cancer, pancreatitis, diabetic retinopathy, or kidney injury should avoid GLP-1s as well. As always, consult with your physician on whether or not GLP-1 medications are appropriate for you.

The cardiovascular benefits of GLP-1 have stirred up excitement in the medical realm too. In a large-sweeping clinical trial known as the SELECT trial, researchers discovered that patients who received GLP-1 doses weekly saw an astonishing 20 percent decrease in cardiovascular events, such as heart attacks and strokes, compared to the placebo group. This improvement was noted in patients who hadn't even lost significant amounts of weight.

There are GLP-1 receptors distributed throughout so many organs and pathways in the body that researchers are just starting to uncover these medications' far-reaching benefits. As of 2024, there are early studies indicating they may be useful in treating lung disease, asthma, colorectal cancer, liver disease, and even neurodegenerative diseases like dementia, to highlight just a few.

GLP-1 medications can also be helpful for people who struggle with food cravings, food addictions, or an unhealthy relationship with food. To an extent, it can alleviate the mental burden of dieting. Working with a licensed therapist is always recommended to address the mental health side of weight loss.

Side Effects and Symptoms

No medication is immune from side effects, and GLP-1 medications can cause a few unpleasant symptoms. The most frequently reported side effects in studies are the following:

- Gastrointestinal complaints: The most common GI symptoms are nausea, diarrhea, bloating, constipation, and vomiting.
- Low blood sugar or blood pressure: Symptoms like dizziness, shakiness, fatigue, sweating, and mood changes are signs of low blood sugar (hypoglycemia) or blood pressure. These symptoms are especially common in patients who are also using medications that can lower blood sugar. If you aren't eating enough calories throughout the day, you will be more prone to crashes.
- Injection site reactions: The most common complaints are redness, itchiness, and swelling, but they are typically mild.

When patients lose weight too quickly, they may experience sagging of the facial skin due to a loss of fat tissue and collagen. This can be reduced by consuming enough calories to ensure that the weight drops at a more moderate pace. It's important to maintain a healthy muscle mass while taking a GLP-1, not only for aesthetic purposes but also for optimal metabolic functioning.

ESSENTIAL

The most important thing you can do to reduce side effects is to stay hydrated. Remind yourself to drink water consistently throughout the day to help with digestion. Sip tea or broth if you're tired of water. Avoid sugary or caffeinated beverages, as they may worsen dehydration. If you do feel dehydrated, eat foods like bananas, avocados, and salty crackers to restore potassium and sodium levels. Dill pickle juice is also a quick fix.

Less common and more extreme side effects of the medication include bowel obstruction, pancreatitis, gastroparesis (paralysis of the stomach), suicidal ideation, and gallstone attacks. Most side effects are not severe, but always consult with your physician if you are concerned about your symptoms.

Helpful Tips for Side Effects

Dealing with side effects from GLP-1 medications can vary depending on the specific symptoms you're experiencing, but here are some general tips:

Nausea

- Eat smaller, more frequent meals.
- Avoid greasy or spicy foods and foods with strong flavors or odors.
- Consume ginger in foods or beverages or in ginger-based supplements.

Diarrhea

- Drink plenty of water.
- Eat foods that are gentle on your stomach, like bananas, rice, applesauce, and toast (BRAT diet).
- If severe, avoid high-fiber foods temporarily.

Gas, bloating, and constipation

- Stay hydrated.
- Eat high-fiber foods, but be mindful of how your body reacts to them. Too much fiber can cause bloating.
- Avoid carbonated beverages.
- Stay physically active.

Low blood sugar (hypoglycemia)

- Always have a source of quick-acting sugar (like glucose tablets or juice) on hand.
- Monitor blood sugar levels regularly if on other diabetes medications.
- If dizziness is due to diarrhea or vomiting, try sipping an electrolyte drink.
- Be sure to fuel your body before and after exercising.

Injection site reactions

- Rotate injection sites and use proper injection techniques.
- Apply a cold pack to the area before injection and massage the site afterward.
- If you notice excessive scarring, it may be an indication of iron deficiency anemia. Boost your iron levels with beans, leafy green vegetables, or red meat.

Working with a team of professionals not only is important for minimizing side effects and reaping the maximum benefits from GLP-1 medications but can also help you eat properly. In extreme cases, you may be prescribed medications to combat the side effects.

Why Is a GLP-1 Diet Important?

Eating while taking a GLP-1 medication is most likely different from your typical diet enjoyed prior to the medication. While on this medication, your appetite and cravings may change, and your hunger signals will likely diminish. It's important to eat well, but it can become more of a complex task.

One of the main concerns from a medical perspective is malnutrition stemming from the fewer calories and nutrients consumed while on the medication. Some patients claim to consume as little as 300 to 500 calories a day for several months. Most major health institutions recommend 1,200 calories a day as a healthy minimum for women and 1,500 calories a day for men. In extreme cases, malnutrition is exacerbated by vomiting and other GI symptoms on the medication.

Although it may sound counterintuitive to be malnourished with a higher BMI, it's a legitimate possibility when you're drastically limiting your calorie intake. Nourishing your body well will give your body the resources it needs to burn fat and get the results you're looking for.

It's important to consume a GLP-1 diet to maintain a healthy metabolism or, put another way, to keep your body burning calories at a healthy rate. When calories dip too low for too long, metabolic adaptation takes place. Metabolic adaptation is your body's way of conserving energy, a protective metabolic process that has evolved from our ancestors. When fewer calories are consumed, your body eventually burns calories more slowly and your overall metabolism decreases. A GLP-1 diet will protect your body's metabolism and fuel it properly for long-term fat burning.

There are also foods and spices you can consume, such as resistant starches and cinnamon, that naturally increase GLP-1 levels and complement the work of the medication. These will be discussed more later in the book.

How Is a GLP-1 Diet Different from Other Diets?

What you've traditionally learned about losing weight is turned upside down on a GLP-1 diet. Your previous eating habits won't work while taking

GLP-1, and you'll need to rethink everything you've learned about losing weight up to this point.

Most traditional weight loss diets focus on limiting your calories and counting exact macronutrients such as protein, fat, and carbohydrates. The idea behind these diets is to restrict your calories enough to stay in a deficit. Although you're going to be watching those same numbers on a GLP-1 diet, you'll be approaching it from the opposite direction.

On GLP-1, the goal is to eat *enough* calories, macronutrients (protein, fat, carbohydrates, and alcohol), and micronutrients (vitamins and minerals) to stay well nourished and maintain a healthy muscle mass and metabolism, while also minimizing side effects as much as possible. To do so, you'll focus on eating smaller, more frequent meals throughout the day to work with your limited appetite. Eating more frequently will help you get the appropriate amount of calories and nutrients you need to keep your body functioning at full capacity. You'll also become more cautious about the foods you can and cannot consume—many people learn this the hard way. Foods that are higher in fats, refined sugars, or spices tend to be rejected. Foods such as lean proteins, vegetables, and fruits tend to be tolerated well. Protein will be a particular focus for maintaining a healthy body composition while losing weight.

Focusing on water is just as important as focusing on the right foods to eat. Weight loss is a driver of dehydration when burning fat. Additionally, water can help facilitate digestion and minimize side effects.

The GLP-1 diet will take time to adjust to both physically and mentally. It's unlike any type of diet you've experienced in the past. Following a GLP-1 diet will be essential for maximizing your weight loss results and minimizing side effects.

CHAPTER 2

Choosing a Healthy GLP-1 Diet

Eating while taking a GLP-1 medication requires a fresh perspective on dieting. Forget everything you know, and approach this with an open mind. You might find yourself eating significantly less than usual, and sometimes, you may not feel hungry at all. Your tastes and tolerances might change, and some of your old favorites might leave you feeling queasy. Navigating this dietary shift without guidance can be challenging and potentially harmful. It's not just about eating smaller portions of your old diet; it's about completely transforming your daily approach to food. This chapter is your guide to understanding the essential principles of eating on GLP-1, crucial for maximizing your results and maintaining long-term weight loss. You'll learn how to calculate your nutritional needs and which macronutrients are the most important in your day-to-day eating plan.

Eating for Weight Loss

Eating for weight loss has never been straightforward. Over the years, the science of healthy eating has evolved dramatically, often presenting contradictory advice that can leave you feeling bewildered. Take eggs, for example. Once shunned as cholesterol villains, they are now hailed as nutrient-rich superfoods. Remember the food pyramid, which once encouraged people to consume 6–11 servings of grains daily? Fast forward to today, and many diet plans advocate for the complete elimination of grains in favor of low-carb alternatives. The constant changes in dietary guidelines can be dizzying. Just as you begin to adapt to one trend, another emerges, turning conventional wisdom on its head. And the introduction of medications like GLP-1s adds another layer of complexity as you try to balance their benefits with potential side effects and lifestyle changes.

The shifting sands of dietary advice can create a lot of confusion. It's not surprising if you feel overwhelmed, not knowing which path to follow. Which recommendations truly support long-term well-being? Which are fads, soon to be replaced by something new? While trends have changed over the years, there are some universal foundations of a well-balanced diet that have stood the test of time:

- Eat a wide variety of different-colored vegetables and fruits every day
- Increase the amount of fiber in your diet (25 grams per day for women up to age 50 or 21 per day over 50; 38 grams per day for men up to age 50 or 30 per day over 50)
- Choose lean, high-quality proteins such as chicken, fish, tofu, beans, and eggs
- Select whole grains, like oatmeal, quinoa, and brown rice
- Consume healthy fats, particularly omega-3s, found in foods like salmon, olive oil, nuts, and seeds
- Enjoy generous servings of herbs and spices in your meals

- Limit ultra-processed foods, especially those high in calories, sodium, and trans fats
- Limit the consumption of alcohol and drinks high in sugar

You may be surprised to see that no specific foods or food groups are eliminated entirely. Contrary to popular diet rhetoric, you can include all foods into a healthy, balanced diet for weight loss. The trick is to take these foundations and make the appropriate modifications for your body and the medication you're taking.

Creating Healthier Habits on GLP-1

Once you start a GLP-1 regimen, you'll quickly recognize the decrease in your appetite. This is a result of delayed gastric emptying. Food now moves through your stomach more slowly. Your body reacts to this by turning your hunger receptors and signaling hormones down. You will find yourself a lot less hungry than you normally are.

ALERT

Mental health is just as important as physical health! Engaging in restrictive dieting can be a significant risk factor for eating disorders, especially for adolescents and young adults. If consuming fewer calories becomes mentally distressing or triggers unhealthy eating behaviors, please talk to your doctor or a mental health professional about your concerns and if the medication is appropriate for you.

While a smaller appetite might sound appealing at first, it's a catch-22. You have to be careful to still consume enough calories, macronutrients (carbohydrates, proteins, and fats), and micronutrients (vitamins and minerals) to nourish your body and provide you with the energy you need. The best way to hit these targets while still honoring your new appetite is to consume smaller meals more frequently throughout the day. For example, you might consume 4–6 small meals throughout the day instead of 2–3 larger meals. This approach can also help by giving you a better variety of nutrients throughout the day. It's also recommended that you eat meals earlier in the day when your insulin response is more efficient and avoid eating large portions within 2–3 hours of going to sleep.

If you experience an extremely low appetite, you may need to set aside time in the day to eat even when you aren't hungry. Give yourself enough time to enjoy your meal slowly so your body has time to digest. You may even graze on a meal over an hour or two if necessary to finish it.

Skipping meals altogether or consuming fewer than 700 calories per day is not safe. It will take time for your body to adapt and find a new rhythm for eating. If you are having trouble consuming an adequate number of calories, we'll discuss tips and tricks for finding palatable food options that are both nutrient and calorie dense later in this chapter. Remember, what you've learned about dieting in the past is turning upside down: Your goal now is to consume enough calories and nutrients throughout the day.

Calculating Your Nutritional Needs

Everyone's exact nutritional needs vary by a variety of factors—no two people have the exact same metabolism or physiology. Here are some of the variables that determine someone's caloric needs:

- **Activity Level:** The more physically active you are, the more calories you need. Activity levels can be categorized as sedentary, moderately active, or very active.
- **Age:** Caloric needs generally decrease with age due to a decline in muscle mass and metabolic rate.
- **Gender:** Males typically have higher caloric needs than females due to greater muscle mass and higher metabolic rate.
- **Body Composition:** Individuals with a higher muscle mass burn more calories at rest compared to those with a higher fat mass.

- **Health Status:** Certain medical conditions, such as COPD or cystic fibrosis, or recovery from an illness can increase caloric needs. Conditions like hypothyroidism can lower them.

Here's a quick formula to help you estimate your target calorie goal while on GLP-1. Take your current weight (in pounds) and multiply it by:

- 13 (if you don't exercise at all)
- 15 (if you exercise a few times weekly)
- 18 (if you exercise five days or more a week)

Voilà! You've calculated your maintenance calorie number. Now you can establish your calorie deficit range. Subtract 500 calories from your maintenance number. This is the higher end of your range. Then, subtract 750 calories from the same maintenance number to establish your lower end. For example, a person who weighs 150 pounds and doesn't exercise at all would need roughly 1,950 calories for maintenance and a calorie deficit range of 1,200–1,450 calories per day. To better understand your specific nutritional needs, working with a registered dietitian can help clarify your goals for weight loss.

Now that you've established an appropriate calorie range, the next step is to determine how those calories are composed. There are four groups (you read that right: not three but *four*!) that can provide your body with calories. They are termed "macronutrients" because they make up a relatively large proportion of what we eat:

Macronutrients and Calories

Macronutrient	Calories	Main Sources
Carbohydrates	4 calories/gram	Vegetables, fruits, grains, breads, legumes
Protein	4 calories/gram	Animal meat, seafood, tofu, dairy, eggs
Fat	9 calories/gram	Oil, avocados, butter, nuts, seeds
Alcohol	7 calories/gram	Wine, beer, cider, vodka, gin

It's traditionally recommended that you get 45–65 percent of your calories from carbohydrates, 10–35 percent from protein, and 20–35 percent from fat. Carbohydrates are the body's primary source of energy, which is why they make up the largest proportion of the recommended diet. They are broken down into glucose, which fuels cells, tissues, and organs, especially the brain and muscles. Protein helps your body build and repair muscle and tissue. Fats are important for hormone building, satiety, and absorption of certain vitamins like A, D, E, and K. For individuals on GLP-1 medications, we are going to tweak the ratios to better complement how the medication works.

Recommended Macronutrient Ratios

Macronutrient	Traditional Ratio	GLP-1 Ratio
Carbohydrates	45%–65%	20%–25%
Protein	10%–35%	30%–40%
Fat	20%–35%	25%–35%
Alcohol	Limited	Limited

Now that we've made it through all of that math, what do these numbers actually look like in your day-to-day life? To translate it simply, you should consume a moderate amount of carbohydrates and fat paired with a higher amount of protein throughout the day.

FACT

An individual food can provide more than one macronutrient. For example, peanuts are made up of carbohydrates, protein, and fat, even though we tend to think of them only as a protein source. We tend to classify foods based on the macronutrient that they are highest in, but most foods are a mix of more than one group.

What Foods to Eat on a GLP-1 Diet

The most common mistake that people make while taking GLP-1 is not consuming enough protein and calories. At the same time, you want to make sure you're not consuming too many carbohydrate-heavy foods, so we will discuss the glycemic index too.

> **ESSENTIAL**
>
> There are many foods that have become popular favorites among GLP-1 users through trial and error. Smaller portions of foods like oatmeal, fruit, or yogurt are great for when you have an upset stomach. If you have trouble digesting red meat, try other protein options like seafood, tofu, or eggs. People who are looking for something sweeter often reach for Italian ice or smoothies.

Protein

Protein is your best friend. Eating higher amounts of protein can increase your lean muscle mass, boost your metabolism, increase your satiety, and promote fat burning. Most notably, protein intake can naturally boost your levels of native GLP-1 hormone, allowing you to enhance the effects of your medication.

Some of the variables that determine the speed of your metabolism—or how quickly your body metabolizes food and burns calories—are out of your control, such as age and genetics. However, there is one variable that plays a significant role in the speed of your metabolism: lean muscle mass. Building more lean muscle mass stems from both exercise and nutrition. Consuming adequate amounts of high-quality protein helps stimulate muscle protein synthesis, which is necessary for building new muscle tissue. While exercise regimens are key to building muscle mass, the nutrition aspect is equally important. You can't out-exercise a poor diet; consistently consuming more calories than you burn will eventually lead to weight gain. Sufficient protein in your diet is essential for muscle repair and maintenance, especially when you're losing weight. Exercise alone without sufficient protein can lead to muscle loss. Plus, a balanced diet helps maintain healthy levels of hormones like insulin and testosterone, which also play important roles in muscle preservation.

Muscle mass is metabolically active, meaning the more lean muscle mass you have, the faster your basal metabolic rate. Since your body requires more energy to break down protein, when you eat foods high in protein, you will be burning more calories throughout the day.

FACT

Basal metabolic rate (BMR) is the number of calories your body needs to maintain basic functions at rest, like breathing, circulating blood, and regulating temperature. Total daily energy expenditure (TDEE), on the other hand, refers to the total amount of calories burned in a day. You may also come across the term NEAT (non-exercise activity thermogenesis), which refers to calories burned through daily activity not classified as exercise, such as climbing the stairs. A nutrition professional will use all of this data to help you calculate your unique calorie deficit number.

When taking GLP-1 medications, it can be extremely challenging to maintain lean muscle mass. The rapid weight loss associated with these medications can result in a higher proportion of muscle loss compared to fat loss. In medical circles, this is referred to as sarcopenia. Here are some signs of sarcopenia:

- You notice less muscle definition
- You feel more fatigued
- Your workout performance or endurance declines
- Your sweat has an ammonia-like odor

Even without these telltale signs of muscle loss, it's still essential to optimize your protein intake. Having a higher muscle mass can also improve your body's response to insulin and soak up more glucose from the bloodstream.

Protein comes in various shapes and forms. The foods most associated with protein are animal meats, but there are many other notable sources out there. Here are some examples of high-protein foods:

- Animal meats
- Seafood
- Eggs
- Cow's milk and soy milk
- Tofu and tempeh
- Protein powder (whey- or plant-based)
- Greek yogurt
- Cheese
- Beans and legumes
- Seeds
- Nuts
- Lentils
- Quinoa

There are simple tips and tricks to sneak in more protein throughout the day. For example, keep a packet of beef jerky or trail mix in your bag for an easy snack. Swap out rice for quinoa, which is higher in protein. Prepare hard-boiled eggs or cooked chickpeas in advance to use as a snack or salad topping later on. Protein powder is a great addition to oatmeal, smoothies, or baked goods.

Calories

While staying in a caloric deficit is a nonnegotiable for weight loss, eating too few calories comes with repercussions as well. Although it's tempting to consume fewer calories to lose more weight, your body has built-in mechanisms to counteract that plan.

Having evolved from our ancestral hunting days, when food sources were scarce for prolonged periods of time, your body will slow down its metabolism to conserve energy. You want to find the sweet spot where you are both burning fat and running your metabolism at top speed.

If you are unsure how many calories you are consuming, try using a calorie counting app (MyFitnessPal is a popular choice) for a few days or a week to determine your baseline intake. It's important to be precise with measurements rather than estimating your intake. Make sure to track on both weekdays and weekends. Some individuals enjoy tracking calories throughout their entire weight loss journey, but it's a personal preference.

If you are not tracking your caloric intake but have concerns that you aren't eating enough, here are some signs that you're consuming too few calories:

- Fatigue
- Mental fog
- Dizziness
- Low blood sugar (hypoglycemia)
- Hair loss
- Feeling cold
- Constipation
- Loss of period
- Weakened immune system

Being under the regular supervision of a doctor and doing routine lab work can also verify whether or not your calories are too low. If you are unable to hit your caloric goal or you're experiencing some of these symptoms, here are tips to increase your calories while still being cognizant of your symptoms:

- Graze on nut-heavy trail mix throughout the day
- Sip on a protein shake with 20–30 grams of protein in a tolerable flavor
- Add whey protein to Greek yogurt, oatmeal, cream cheese, or pancake mix
- Add avocado slices or a hard-cooked egg to a snack or salad
- Use generous amounts of cooking oils

Remember, eating small meals more frequently throughout the day will be easier than consuming larger meals. For instance, if your goal is to consume 1,200 calories a day, consider breaking that into six small meals or snacks around 200 calories. You might find it helpful to set alarms or reminders on your phone to make sure you eat enough.

If your nausea or symptoms are too extreme to eat an adequate amount of food for prolonged periods, consult with your doctor about the appropriateness of your dose or type of medication. It's important to find the medication that is right for you.

Lower–Glycemic Index Foods

The glycemic index (GI) can be helpful in finding the best carbohydrate sources for maintaining stable blood sugar. The GI was developed in the 1980s to rank carbohydrate sources based on how much they make your blood sugar rise after eating. Foods are ranked on a 1–100 scale, with lower scores indicating the smallest rise in blood sugar.

Lower-GI foods include apples, pears, berries, cherries, peaches, grapefruit, beans, legumes, non-starchy vegetables, wild rice, wheat pasta, and steel cut oats. These foods take longer to digest than higher-GI foods. They cause a smaller rise in blood glucose, which helps prevent a spike in insulin as well.

Moderating your carbohydrate and sugar intake will help GLP-1 medications work most effectively. By choosing more low-GI foods, you'll find you're eating more produce, beans and legumes, and whole grains, instead of the more processed foods that tend to have a higher GI score. It's easy to incorporate low-GI foods into your diet. Here are a few options to try:

- Greek yogurt with berries and chia seeds
- Hummus with cucumbers or celery
- Apple slices with nut butter
- Cottage cheese with peaches
- Lentil salad with cucumber and red onion

Foods Not to Eat on GLP-1

You may have already learned through trial and error that certain foods don't agree with you while you're on the medication. Whether they are simply no longer palatable or cause legitimate side effects such as bloating, diarrhea, acid reflux, or nausea, there are foods you'll want to steer clear of while taking the medication.

Think of eating on GLP-1 as if you were eating for an upset stomach. Many of the same principles apply, since GLP-1 affects the motility and functionality of the gastrointestinal tract. The main two categories of foods to avoid are greasy, low-quality fat sources and foods high in refined sugars or carbohydrates. Even on low doses of the medication, these two groups of food can be hard to tolerate.

Coincidentally, these are also foods that can have negative impacts on your health when consumed excessively, so learning to minimize them will be helpful for your health in the long run. Let's dive into each of these groups.

Poor-Quality Fats

High-fat foods can exacerbate the gastrointestinal side effects of the medication. However, you should not avoid *all* fats. The human body doesn't produce fats; you need to consume them so they can be used in your body's production of hormones, vitamins, and cholesterol, among other things. Healthy, anti-inflammatory fats, such as omega-3s, are beneficial on a GLP-1 diet, especially when you're looking for ways to increase your calories. You want to increase the healthy sources of fat and minimize the poor-quality ones.

QUESTION

What is the Mediterranean diet?

The Mediterranean diet is a popular and research-backed eating pattern modeled after the traditional diets of countries bordering the Mediterranean Sea. The diet emphasizes whole foods like fruits, vegetables, whole grains, and healthy fats such as olive oil. It includes moderate consumption of fish, poultry, and dairy, with limited red meat. This heart-healthy lifestyle consistently receives the title #1 Best Diet Overall from *US News & World Report*.

Fats are categorized by their structure: monounsaturated, polyunsaturated, saturated, and trans fats. Here are examples of foods that contain each type:

- **Monounsaturated fats:** Nuts, seeds, avocados, olive oil, canola oil, dark chocolate
- **Polyunsaturated fats (omega-3s and omega-6s):** Fish, walnuts, seeds
- **Saturated fats:** Animal meats, butter, cheese, dairy products, coconut oil, mayonnaise
- **Trans fats:** Fast food, cakes, shortening

Monounsaturated and polyunsaturated fats have the most evidence linking them to positive health benefits, such as lowering the "bad" cholesterol, while trans fats are most harmful for your health. When consuming fats on a GLP-1 diet, focus on the monounsaturated and polyunsaturated sources just mentioned.

If you consume saturated fats, focus on high-quality sources (such as pasture-raised eggs, grass-fed beef, or wild-caught fish) in moderate amounts, as high intakes of saturated fats are associated with gastrointestinal symptoms.

Here are some examples of high-fat foods to limit:

- French fries
- Onion rings
- Fatty cuts of meat, such as pork belly
- Fried meats, such as fried chicken
- Poultry skin
- Potato chips
- Pork bacon
- Doughnuts

It takes the body longer to digest fats compared to other macronutrients such as protein and carbohydrates. Fats are not water-soluble, so the body has to produce specialized enzymes to break them down. High-fat foods also slow down the emptying of the stomach, compounding the effect of GLP-1. When food sits in the digestive tract too long, this pulls in more water, leading to bloating, nausea, and diarrhea. Your body will quickly communicate to you which types of fatty foods are off-limits.

Refined Carbohydrates

Another category of foods that can cause unwanted side effects is refined carbohydrates. Refined carbohydrates are carbohydrates that are stripped down to their basic form, wiping out many beneficial nutrients, including fiber, vitamins, minerals, and antioxidants. Your body digests and converts refined carbohydrates into blood sugar more rapidly. Consequently, your blood sugar level spikes quickly and your body is forced to release extra insulin.

You are likely familiar with foods that are classified as refined carbohydrates. These foods include white flour, white bread, white rice, pastries, sodas, pasta, sweets, breakfast cereals, and added sugars. Typically, these foods are very high in carbohydrates and can also be high in added sugar. Reading nutrition labels will help you determine what is an appropriate choice. If you're eating out, check the menu or website ahead of time to find the nutrition information. Aim for under 40 grams of carbohydrates in your main meals and under 30 grams of carbohydrates in your snacks or desserts.

When searching for healthier carbohydrate options, look for foods or labels that include whole grains or some fiber. The daily recommendation for fiber is 25 grams per day for women and 38 grams per day for men (the current average intake in the United States is 15 grams). Some examples of these foods include brown rice, beans, lentils, bran cereal, barley, couscous, chickpeas, sweet potatoes, carrots, and steel cut oats. A helpful tip when it comes to fiber is the 10:1 rule: Choose foods where for every 10 grams of carbohydrates, there is 1 gram of fiber.

ESSENTIAL

If you're having trouble switching from white grains to whole-grain products, try mixing half of each to start. For example, blend half white rice and half brown rice. You won't notice a huge difference in the taste.

Fiber is also fantastic for maintaining a healthy gut microbiome—the diverse community of microorganisms, including bacteria, viruses, fungi, and other microbes, that inhabit the gastrointestinal tract. Fiber promotes satiety and healthy bowel movements and helps to lower cholesterol, balance hormones, and reduce the risk of colon cancer. It's a powerhouse nutrient all around.

However, consuming foods with very high fiber can distress the gut, especially if you don't regularly consume lots of fiber. Some users notice problems with more fibrous, cruciferous foods such as broccoli, cabbage, or cauliflower.

Drink Precautions

Alcohol can work against the mechanisms of GLP-1. For example, alcohol inhibits the body's process of producing glucose and releasing insulin, which can increase the risk of hypoglycemia (low blood sugar). Alcohol speeds up the emptying of the stomach, while GLP-1 slows it down. In short, GLP-1 works to balance blood sugar and alcohol disrupts it. These conflicting metabolic processes can cause unpredictable blood sugar swings and exacerbate symptoms like nausea, vomiting, and dehydration.

FACT

A standard alcoholic drink contains about 14 grams of pure alcohol. A standard drink is 12 ounces of beer (5% alcohol), 5 ounces of wine (12% alcohol), or 1.5 ounces of distilled spirits like vodka or whiskey (40% alcohol). Understanding standard drink sizes helps track alcohol consumption and reduces the risk of overconsumption or related health issues.

And remember that alcohol can suppress hunger. Since medications like GLP-1 already reduce appetite, it's important not to further amplify that side effect. If you are going to consume alcohol, limit yourself to 1–2 standard drinks in one day, and pair them with meals.

When selecting an alcoholic drink, avoid sugary mixed drinks. Choose lower-carbohydrate drinks like dry wine, light beer, or a low–alcohol by volume (ABV) drink such as a wine spritzer. And it's a good idea to wait at least 24 hours after your weekly dose of the medication before consuming any alcohol.

Coincidentally, many people report drinking less alcohol on the medication thanks to fewer cravings and curbed addictions. Patients and doctors have also noted fewer urges for nicotine and opioids. The brain mechanisms responsible for overeating overlap with the mechanisms responsible for addictions. The GLP-1 hormone may reduce the dopamine rush that is commonly reported from that first sip of alcohol or first bite of cake.

Other beverages that can lead to side effects like burping, bloating, or indigestion include caffeine and carbonated drinks. To avoid these issues, consider drinking more water, as it can help boost your metabolism and support digestion.

Spicy Foods

Chilies and other spicy foods contain a mix of acids and a compound called capsaicin, which binds to pain receptors from the mouth through the gastrointestinal tract. The acids can also irritate the stomach lining, resulting in the familiar burning sensation. When the gastrointestinal tract is moving slower, reactions like this can feel prolonged and more intense.

> **FACT**
>
> Spices like ginger and turmeric are excellent additions to smoothies, main dishes, and desserts, as they help reduce inflammation and ease nausea. Consider trying ginger tea, sprinkling ginger into stir-fries, or even adding it to a trail mix. Turmeric is often used in golden milk, curries, dips, smoothies, and egg dishes.

Just be mindful not to force any particular foods on your body. Even though you've enjoyed these foods in the past, what your body can tolerate changes while on the medication. It will take time to learn what your body can digest, and this is a golden opportunity to truly understand your body's signals and feedback.

Consider keeping a food journal that logs foods eaten along with symptoms to pick up on any patterns your body is trying to communicate. Every individual will have a unique reaction to the medication—this is your personal journey to explore!

CHAPTER 3

Creating Healthy Habits

Many people view GLP-1 medications as "miracle drugs," but it's misleading to assume they work without any effort. In fact, this couldn't be further from the truth. The long-term effectiveness of GLP-1 medication depends on making diet and lifestyle changes to support it. Unfortunately, many people fall into the trap of believing that this "miracle" medication is a quick fix for weight loss. While it may yield impressive short-term results, long-term success necessitates essential dietary and lifestyle changes.

For those who stop taking GLP-1 abruptly, whether due to changes in insurance coverage or other reasons, the weight often begins to return. In one study, individuals who stopped taking GLP-1 and abandoned lifestyle changes regained two-thirds of their lost weight within a year. Additionally, cardio-metabolic improvements, such as improved cholesterol or blood pressure, also reversed. It's crucial to remember that this class of medication is a treatment, not a cure. To achieve the best results both during and after using GLP-1, fundamental dietary and lifestyle changes that support weight loss and overall health are essential.

Don't Forget about Water!

While hydration is necessary on a day-to-day basis for survival, it serves many more functions than that. For weight loss specifically, staying hydrated promotes the body's fat-burning mechanisms. The physiological term for burning fat is "lipolysis." *Lipo* means "fat" and *lysis* means "breaking apart." The first step in lipolysis is breaking up the fatty triglyceride chains using water molecules. To keep things in simple terms: Without water, the body cannot properly metabolize fat. Even mild dehydration can slow down this process. Unsurprisingly, some users have noticed more accelerated weight loss on days when they are most hydrated.

Digestion is another critical process that relies on drinking plenty of water. Good hydration supports the body's production of digestive juices, such as saliva, stomach acid, and other enzymes. GLP-1 medications slow the pace of digestion, but drinking sufficient water can help keep your gastrointestinal tract moving along smoothly. Dehydration can exacerbate GLP-1 side effects like constipation, nausea, fatigue, and bloating. In extreme cases of dehydration, there's also a risk for kidney infections, gallstones, or muscle cramps. If you're already experiencing nausea or diarrhea, the need for water is even more critical to replenish the fluids lost.

ESSENTIAL

Take advantage of reminders and tools that can help you stay better hydrated. Set phone alarms or use hydration apps like Plant Nanny, WaterMinder, Hydro Coach, or Aqualert to encourage frequent water intake.

It can be tricky to stay sufficiently hydrated. Your stomach empties slower and you feel fuller than you normally would—and this applies to hydration too. You might not recognize thirst in the same way you're accustomed to. You might even notice that water has a different "taste," which can make it harder to consume enough.

Here are a few ideas on how to get more water throughout the day:

- Infuse water with herbs or sliced fruits or vegetables (like mint, lemon, or cucumber) to enhance the flavor.
- Carry your favorite water bottle around with you through the day.
- Drink water through a straw to encourage quicker sipping.
- Incorporate foods with high water content, like soups and broths, into your diet.
- Pair drinking water with other habits, such as driving to work or sending an email.
- Water down drinks such as juices, iced teas, or sports drinks.
- Minimize coffee, energy drinks, and alcohol, as they have diuretic effects.

So, what's the appropriate amount to consume? General recommendations say around 2–3 liters of water per day, but this is subject to a variety of personal factors, such as body weight, activity level, age, and your climate. It's best to adjust your intake so that your urine remains pale or clear by the end of the day (urine is most concentrated first thing in the morning). You might also want to bump up your water intake more if you sweat heavily, have vomiting or diarrhea, or notice other signs of dehydration. If you're having these symptoms or constantly struggling to get enough water in general, consider adding in electrolytes for optimal hydration.

Get Enough Sleep

A healthy amount of sleep, usually between 7 and 9 hours a night, is one of the most overlooked tools for weight loss. Inadequate sleep is considered a stand-alone risk factor for obesity. There is a clear connection indicating that individuals who sleep less than 7 hours a night are more likely to have a high BMI. It's also considered a risk factor for poor cardiovascular and metabolic health, type 2 diabetes, and even premature death.

When you're sleep-deprived, many of your internal processes are thrown off-kilter. On a metabolic level, lack of sleep causes your body's insulin responsiveness to drop within just a few days. Researchers discovered that within just four days of inadequate sleep, your body's insulin response can decline up to 30 percent. Remember, when your body isn't properly responding to insulin, you're going to store more glucose as fat. A lack of sleep can spike cortisol, which also cues your body to store fat. In addition, your levels of ghrelin, the hunger hormone, will rise (you become hungrier), while you also experience a drop in leptin, the satiety hormone (you become less full).

Sleep-deprived individuals are also more likely to make poor food choices. Let's be honest. Who is reaching for a salad at 2 a.m.? Sleeping less can sabotage your weight loss efforts and hard-earned results. Here are a few practical steps to take for better sleep:

- Maintain a regular sleep schedule. Try to wake up and go to bed at the same time every day, even on the weekends. Make sure you are getting natural sunlight exposure throughout the day to reset your circadian rhythm.
- Create a comfortable, cool, dark, and quiet sleep environment. Invest in a good mattress and pillows. Use an eye mask or a white noise machine if needed.
- Create a relaxing bedtime routine. Wind down with calming activities like reading or taking a warm bath. Avoid electronic devices at bedtime. They emit blue light, which interferes with melatonin production, making it harder to fall asleep.
- Avoid stimulants like caffeine later in the day. Alcohol can disrupt sleep as well.
- Get regular exercise during the day, but avoid exercising vigorously right before bedtime.
- Aim for at least 30 minutes of moderate exercise a day.
- Practice relaxation techniques like deep breathing or meditation to reduce presleep stress.

- Try not to nap during the day. If you do need a nap, keep it to no more than 30 minutes.
- Monitor the quality of your sleep. Keep a sleep journal or use a sleep tracking device to monitor your sleep cycles and identify patterns or issues. This can help you make adjustments.

Unfortunately, it can be difficult to maintain good sleep while you're taking a GLP-1 medication. According to a study published in 2023, sleep interruptions were a common side effect of GLP-1, alongside anxiety and depression—which can also impair sleep. Yet some users have noticed improvements in sleep apnea, insomnia, and other sleep-related conditions on GLP-1. These conflicting reports are not surprising. Sleep and eating overlap, physiologically speaking. When you manipulate one, you also disrupt the other. If the medication is noticeably and consistently impairing your ability to sleep, consult your healthcare professional for solutions.

Manage Your Stress Level

Excessive, chronic stress is just as detrimental to your weight loss journey as inadequate sleep; both can significantly hinder your weight loss efforts. The body's stress mechanisms stem from our ancestors but haven't fully adapted to our modern environment. Even though we are no longer running from predators, our body still initiates the same mechanisms for modern stressors.

When your body is under stress, it shifts toward retaining calories and storing fat as a protective mechanism. Your body doesn't know when the stressor will end—even if *you* know that the work deadline is just a few days away. Your body also pumps out extra cortisol, the fight-or-flight hormone, which compounds the fat storing. Plus, high cortisol can ramp up hunger hormones. In short, a stressed-out body can counteract the work of GLP-1.

Minimizing stress doesn't have a one-size-fits-all solution; it involves two key approaches: reducing stressors (minimizing input) and boosting stress relievers (maximizing output). Stressors can include work, family, finances, or significant life events, while stress relievers may include practices like meditation, therapy, journaling, physical activity, quality sleep, and time spent outdoors. Everyone operates with a different tolerance and threshold for stress in their life as well.

FACT

A high cortisol level can lead to negative effects all over the body. It can impair cognitive function, resulting in difficulty concentrating and memory problems. Additionally, elevated cortisol can weaken the immune system, making you more susceptible to infections and illnesses, and can disrupt sleep patterns, contributing to insomnia.

For some people, reducing stress could look like setting better boundaries for work-life balance. For other people, it could be eliminating unhealthy sources of stress in their life, such as a toxic relationship. Finding hobbies you love can also be a great way to distract and relax your mind! If you're constantly feeling like you are under a high level of stress, consider working with a mental health therapist to find helpful solutions for coping.

Make Strength Training a Regular Habit

Exercise, specifically strength training, is a nonnegotiable habit on GLP-1. Pairing the medication with an appropriate training regimen can enhance insulin sensitivity, promote fat burning, improve sleep, and boost the overall effectiveness of the GLP-1 hormone.

While prescribing a specific exercise regimen is outside the scope of this book, it's impossible to stress enough the importance of strength training. Individuals using GLP-1 are at a high risk of losing muscle mass because of the nature of rapid weight loss. For older or post-menopausal women taking the medication, the risks are even greater. These groups are already at risk for bone fragility or osteoporosis and, ultimately, falls and injuries. It's important to remember that weight loss doesn't automatically equate to a healthier body. The composition of that body weight is equally important.

One of the best ways to combat this change in composition is through consistent strength training. Strength training, also referred to as resistance training, is a form of exercise designed to improve muscular strength and endurance. It involves performing exercises that target specific muscle groups using various forms of resistance, such as free weights, resistance bands, or body weight. Strength training does contribute to fat loss, but indirectly. When you lift an amount of weight that uses close to a muscle's maximum effort, glycogen stores in the muscles become depleted. This prepares the muscles to absorb more glucose during your next meal. This repeated process trains the body to direct more carbohydrates into muscle tissue rather than being stored as fat. Building more muscle mass also increases your metabolic rate, creating a win-win scenario.

Researchers suggest at least two days of resistance training per week, with an increase to three to four days being even more beneficial. If you're newer to strength training, here are a few ways to get started:

- If you don't have access to a gym, you can still perform calisthenic exercises at home, such as push-ups, dips, pull-ups, and bodyweight squats. These exercises can be progressively intensified by adding weights over time.
- If you're low on time, try incorporating exercise snacks: short bouts of high-repetition exercises performed with minimal to no equipment, repeated throughout the day or week. For example, you might do fifteen chair squats as a quick and effective workout.
- If you need more guidance, apps like StrongLifts or Fitbod can generate personalized strength training workouts based on your fitness level and equipment available. *Barbell Medicine Podcast* is a great resource for more education on the topic.

Make sure to increase your calories in tandem with your workouts, since burning extra calories through exercise can drop your calorie deficit dangerously low.

Avoid Nutrient Deficiencies

When you consume fewer calories, you also consume fewer vitamins, minerals, and other essential nutrients. Malnutrition has become a growing topic of concern within the community of GLP-1 prescribers and users. If you eat non-nutrient-dense foods, just in smaller portions, you may become malnourished and metabolically unhealthy. Think of every meal as a critical opportunity to fuel your body and pack in as many nutrients as possible.

While nutrient deficiencies aren't always something you can "feel" as a symptom, your body, especially your fat-burning pathways, will not be running at full capacity without the nutrients it needs. It's the equivalent of your car running with bad oil in the engine. It's not always something you notice right away, but it can wreak havoc in the long run.

Similar to what's seen in bariatric surgery, reducing intake and impairing the digestion process over time can lead to dangerous nutrient deficiencies. In a study done on Japanese patients who had both bariatric surgery and subsequent semaglutide injections, researchers uncovered deficiencies in B12, zinc, albumin, and skeletal muscle. From this list, vitamin B12 is the most commonly noted deficiency, and for good reason. The body absorbs vitamin B12 through the stomach during digestion. When stomach emptying is delayed, as it is with GLP-1, vitamin B12 doesn't get absorbed as effectively as it should.

B12 is one of the most helpful vitamins for weight loss, energy, and metabolism, so if you find yourself feeling abnormally fatigued after starting a GLP-1 medication, it might be due to a deficiency in this particular vitamin. Vitamin B12 also helps prevent anemia, a blood condition that can make you feel constantly tired. It's so integral to our fat-burning processes that some studies have suggested B12 deficiency as a stand-alone risk factor for type 2 diabetes and obesity.

Even outside of GLP-1 medications, B vitamin levels are chronically low in the US population. Some estimates suggest that up to one-fifth of the population has marginal deficiency of B12.

Vitamin B12 is naturally found in eggs, poultry, fish, and dairy, but it can also be supplemented via injection, pill, or powder. Women, in particular, should take a broad-spectrum B-vitamin complex to cover other common B-vitamin deficiencies related to hormone fluctuations and birth control.

ESSENTIAL

Snacks rich in vitamin B12 include cheese, boiled eggs, and Greek yogurt. For a quick boost, try tuna or salmon in snack-sized portions. Fortified cereals and nutritional yeast are excellent plant-based options for vegans. Beef jerky is also an excellent source for a convenient, on-the-go B12 snack.

Iron is another important nutrient to monitor while on the medication. A study in the *Journal of Clinical Endocrinology & Metabolism* found a decline in hematocrit and hemoglobin levels after just six months of medication therapy. This decrease may be attributed to reduced stomach acid, which is necessary for the absorption of iron in the duodenum (the first part of the small intestine). It can also be attributed to consuming lower amounts of iron-rich foods, such as red meat. Frequent lab work will be important for monitoring iron levels.

Other common nutrients where deficiencies may occur while on the medication include calcium, zinc, and vitamin D.

While it's always best to get our nutrients from food, supplementation should be a strong consideration for people who reduce their food intake. Here are a few other supplements you might want to take to maximize your weight loss results:

- **Vitamin D:** Improves inflammation and insulin sensitivity and suppresses fat storage
- **Omega-3 fatty acids:** Improves inflammation and insulin sensitivity
- **Chromium:** Assists with insulin sensitivity and regulating appetite
- **Probiotics:** Cultivates healthy gut microbiome and digestion

If you're unsure about which supplements to take, a well-rounded multivitamin is always a great place to start. Work with your medical team to figure out the best supplementation plan for you.

Start a Healthy Relationship with Food

While many physical changes take place in your body on GLP-1, there are mental adaptations happening too, especially in areas related to food intake, energy balance, and even cognitive function. While researchers are still working to learn how synthetic GLP-1 interacts with the brain and how it manages to cross the blood-brain barrier—something that larger molecules like itself typically cannot do—it's crucial to maintain a healthy approach to eating.

QUESTION

What's the difference between eating disorders and disordered eating?

Eating disorders are severe mental health conditions that are diagnosable and require professional treatment, such as anorexia nervosa or binge eating disorder. In contrast, disordered eating encompasses a range of irregular eating behaviors that may not meet the full criteria for an eating disorder, such as feeling guilty after certain food choices, emotional eating, overexercising, or skipping meals.

For many people who have been on the diet roller coaster for years, an unhealthy relationship with food is often the by-product. Whether that comes from strict calorie counting, being taught to avoid certain "bad" foods, binging foods after a diet, or using food as a coping mechanism, an unhealthy relationship with food can exist on a broad spectrum. It can range from almost constant dieting to an extreme obsession or fixation around food and body image.

There's no doubt that food is deeply intertwined with our emotions and culture. It can act as a centerpiece for celebrations or social gatherings. A specific food can be a reminder of happy childhood memories. The art of scratch cooking and baking is therapeutic or cathartic for many. It's nearly impossible to have a neutral relationship with food, but it is possible to have a healthy one.

When you minimize the amount of food you eat, it's important to do so in a way that protects your mental health. The most common trap to fall into is the binge-restrict cycle. Restricting any type of specific food or food group can set you up for a rebound "binge" episode. If you follow an eating plan that completely cuts out your favorite food, whether it's bread, chocolate, or ice cream, it's hard to stop thinking about it.

ESSENTIAL

Ways to honor your body include listening to your body's hunger and fullness cues, eating without distractions, and enjoying your meals mindfully. Focus on whole, nutritious foods, but allow for indulgences without guilt. Consider whether you're eating for physical hunger or emotional reasons. Journaling can help you identify emotional triggers.

Since you're already decreasing your calories, it's important not to restrict foods any further than necessary to manage side effects. Instead, a healthy, sustainable weight loss approach incorporates all foods and food groups. Your body will certainly respond to some foods better than others, but banning any one food will most likely backfire.

A healthy relationship with food also includes honoring and responding to your body's hunger and satiety signals. While hunger can be suppressed while taking the medication, do your best to still respond to your natural cues. If you don't feel any hunger signals at all, try setting up scheduled times throughout the day to eat a small snack or meal. Sometimes eating a small amount can stimulate your hunger hormones.

If your hunger is so suppressed that you are consuming less than 500–700 calories per day, speak to your physician about your dosing and type of medication. If you have a history of eating disorders or disordered eating, speak to your team about whether the treatment is appropriate for you.

Other Tips and Tricks for Staying Healthy on GLP-1

The more tools you have in your toolbox on your weight loss journey, the better. The most effective step you can take on your GLP-1 journey is to educate yourself and build a collection of tools, from helpful technology to supportive friends and a comprehensive care team. As we are still at the forefront of understanding GLP-1 medications, it's important to continue exploring the research and resources that are emerging all the time.

Meal Planning

Meal planning should be a weekly routine for anyone, whether you're on a weight loss journey or not. Not only does it help you stay on track with healthier choices throughout the week, it's also a helpful tool for budgeting and minimizing food waste.

We all have experienced the scenario of the day going differently than we expected, running out of time to cook a meal, and instead driving through the fast-food line to grab something in a pinch. While you can't avoid this scenario completely, having meals or ingredients planned ahead of time can certainly help to prepare you for the unexpected. Ironically, for those with the busiest schedules, prepping meals just one day a week can save more time in the long run than eating out.

Meal planning is not only a time-saving strategy; according to a 2017 French nutritional study, it's also associated with healthier BMIs. In this study, researchers gathered data from participants regarding their meal planning, dietary quality, food variety, weight, and height. They compared these factors to meal planning. It was found that individuals who planned meals were more likely to have better diet quality and variety. Among women, meal planning was associated with lower odds of overweight or obesity.

While prepping all of your meals ahead on one day of the week is the most efficient method, there's no right or wrong way to go about meal planning. It can be as simple as planning out a few meals for your week or as complicated as prepping the whole week's meals on a Sunday. Most people find a balance somewhere in between.

ESSENTIAL

Invest in good-quality containers for meal prep. Use airtight glass containers for storing meals. They're durable, eco-friendly, and microwave-safe. For portion control, opt for BPA-free plastic or silicone containers with dividers. Stackable containers help maximize fridge space, keeping meals fresh and organized throughout the week.

If you're completely new to meal planning, start small. For example, you could double each recipe that you're already planning to cook throughout the week, then either eat the extra servings as leftovers or freeze them for later. Maximizing each cooking opportunity with more servings will cut down on your cooking time dramatically.

If you want to take it a step further, try prepping some snacks, easy breakfasts, or protein sources on the weekend to enjoy the rest of the week. Figure out where your weakest link is and prepare for that. For example, if you have trouble hitting your protein goal, prepare a few ready-to-go high-protein snacks like hard-boiled eggs or turkey roll-ups. If breakfast is always a challenge for you, cook some egg bites or breakfast casseroles ahead of time. The good news is that most of the recipes in this book can be prepared in advance and stored for later.

If you want to maximize your meal prep, choose one or two days each week to spend a few hours in the kitchen preparing several meals at once.

Sunday is a traditionally popular day for meal prepping, but picking a second day mid-week will keep your meals fresher. To make it more enjoyable, invite some friends over and prep your meals together!

Meal Timing

Meal timing is a lesser-known strategy for keeping your blood sugar in check, but an equally important concept to understand. Although your body usually runs like a well-oiled machine, you are, in fact, not a robot. Your hormones are fluctuating constantly throughout the day, mostly unbeknownst to you. A classic example of this is the sleep hormone melatonin. Your melatonin levels peak when darkness sets in and gradually decrease throughout the night as you sleep until they hit their lowest point at wakening.

QUESTION

What is a continuous glucose monitor?

Continuous glucose monitors (CGMs) are wearable devices that track blood sugar levels in real time. A small sensor placed under the skin measures glucose levels throughout the day, providing continuous data to a linked device or app. CGMs help individuals monitor and manage their blood sugar more effectively, offering insights to prevent spikes or drops.

The cycle of one hormone is particularly important for anyone taking GLP-1: insulin. Remember, insulin is the hormone that helps your cells take in glucose (sugar) from the bloodstream to be used for energy. People can experience a condition known as insulin resistance when their cells do not respond effectively to insulin. As a result, their body pumps out more insulin to overcome the resistance. Higher levels of circulating insulin can lead to more weight gain.

There are two ways that intentional meal timing can combat insulin resistance. First, eating smaller meals more frequently throughout the day can lower your body's insulin response. It's most likely this will be your eating pattern already if you're experiencing a reduced appetite. Second, your body is more insulin sensitive in the morning and less in the evening. Eating a substantial breakfast and a smaller dinner meal will work with, rather than against, your body's natural rhythms.

If you're curious to learn more about your blood sugar balance throughout the day, consider using a one-time finger-stick glucose test or a continuous glucose monitor (CGM) to get more personalized data.

Building a Support Network

One of the most underrated keys for success is having both a personal and a professional team to support you. While GLP-1 medications may offer rapid weight loss results, long-term success is rarely something people can achieve on their own. Friends and family provide essential emotional support, encouragement, and even practical help, such as being a gym buddy or meal prep partner. Connecting with others on a similar weight loss journey can also be incredibly motivating.

On top of your personal support network, here are a few of the professionals you could consider bringing onto your team:

- Your prescribing physician
- Registered dietitian
- Mental health therapist
- Health coach or accountability coach
- Personal trainer or fitness instructor
- Physical therapist/chiropractor
- GLP-1 support group

Seek out professionals experienced with weight loss or, specifically, GLP-1 medications. There's no need to feel guilty or embarrassed about seeking professional help. Learning on your own can go a long way, but professional experts can accelerate the learning curve. Just remember that you don't have to figure this out on your own!

CHAPTER 4

Maintaining Weight Loss

How can you maintain long-term weight loss? To lose weight and keep it off, you will need to consistently address both the metabolic aspect of weight loss and the nutritional component. GLP-1 medications are effective at enhancing the body's metabolic response, but this is just one aspect of a broader lifelong weight loss and maintenance journey. They are marketed as a lifelong medication, but many people are either not interested in long-term use or may not have the resources to commit to it. In fact, according to insurance claims data, 85 percent of people who started taking Ozempic stopped taking it within two years, and 71 percent stopped within one year. This chapter explores key principles of sustainable weight loss and the future of medical weight loss therapies.

Hitting a Plateau

While many people taking a GLP-1 medication experience the seemingly instantaneous weight loss that's been popularized in the news and on social media, there's also a group for whom the medication doesn't work at all or stops working after a period of using it. It's estimated that 10–15 percent of patients may not experience significant weight loss or may not respond to the medication at all, according to a 2021 study in the *New England Journal of Medicine.*

Although there are many stories circulating about extremely rapid weight loss, that shouldn't be your goal. A healthy target to aim for is a weight loss of 0.5–2 pounds per week, depending on your starting weight. If you have a higher starting weight, you may achieve losses at the upper end of that range. At this trajectory, you can still safely maintain muscle mass and body composition. Don't compare your experience to that of someone you read about or see online. Losing weight at a rate of half a pound a week or 1 pound every two weeks is not a plateau. It's actually a healthy rate.

For some people, weight loss does slow down or even stop. One of the most dangerous approaches when hitting a weight loss plateau is to double down on the intensity. This is true for any type of diet. You may want to cut calories even more or go to the gym more often. When you're taking a GLP-1 medication, it may even be tempting to ask your doctor to increase the dosage to break through a plateau. But more often than not, this isn't the solution.

When weight loss slows or stops on a GLP-1 medication, it can be due to a combination of physiological adaptation, lifestyle factors, and emotional issues. Here are just a few possible physical blocks:

- **Your caloric intake may have changed.** Even though your appetite has decreased, you may be consuming too many calories if you slowly increase portion sizes or the number of daily snacks. If you're consuming too few calories, your metabolism may slow down and signal your body to conserve fat stores. Adjusting your intake slightly can often jumpstart progress.

- **You may be losing muscle mass.** When weight loss includes muscle loss, your metabolism is decreased. You may need to increase your physical activity, particularly strength or resistance training.
- **Your dosage may be incorrect.** Repeatedly missing doses can cause weight gain. Be sure to take the medication on a regular schedule. You may also need a change in dosage or the type of medication, so check in with your medical care provider.

Keep in mind that other metrics, such as waist circumference, clothing size, or body fat composition may still change, even if your weight stays the same.

ESSENTIAL

Stanford psychologist Carol Dweck popularized the concept of fixed and growth mindsets in her 2006 book, *Mindset: The New Psychology of Success.* People with a fixed mindset believe that certain qualities are innate and unchangeable. For example, someone with a fixed mindset might believe they're not good at a particular skill and that they'll never improve. People with this mindset often stay within their comfort zones and tend to abandon tasks when faced with failure. Someone with a growth mindset understands that while they may not be skilled at something yet, they have the ability to learn, grow, and improve over time. People with this mindset will be more successful with their weight loss and other goals in life.

You might also run into mental blocks. Here are a few examples:

- **Fear of failure:** Worrying about not achieving goals can prevent you from starting or continuing your efforts. If you've had bad experiences with dieting in the past, it may be connected to this common mental block.

- **All-or-nothing thinking:** Viewing success in black-and-white terms can cause you to give up if you slip up once.
- **Comparison with others:** Constantly comparing your journey to others' can lead to feelings of inadequacy or frustration.
- **Emotional attachment to food:** Using food as a source of comfort or reward can create a barrier to making healthier choices.
- **Fear of change:** Worrying about how weight loss will impact your relationships or lifestyle can create resistance to change. For example, you might feel that you can no longer enjoy the same restaurants or social events with your friends.

Weight loss is just as much of a mental game as it is a physical one. Take a step back to evaluate where your barriers may lie.

Why Is Long-Term Weight Loss So Difficult?

The flaw in many weight loss approaches, including GLP-1 treatment, is the lack of sustained weight loss. Studies have repeatedly shown that diets fail. In fact, various studies suggest that 80–95 percent of diets result in weight regain within a few years, and 23 percent end up at a higher weight than their original starting point. Because of this high failure rate, the average person attempts 4–6 diets over their lifetime. These statistics highlight the fact that most diets aren't designed for long-term weight loss. Although there isn't one specific culprit, here are a few reasons why most diet plans don't result in sustained weight loss:

- **An overemphasis on a quick fix:** When people expect quick results, they can become discouraged and give up prematurely.
- **Unrealistic expectations:** A healthy amount of weight loss is estimated to be between 1 and 2 pounds per week, but many people abandon a weight loss plan when they don't experience a massive drop in weight.
- **Lack of support or accountability:** Weight loss should not be a solo journey. Research shows that individuals with strong external

support—such as friends, family, or weight loss peers—tend to achieve more lasting results than those who go it alone.

- **Lack of education or professional guidance:** Weight loss is a complex process, so having the right experts, such as medical professionals, nutritionists, therapists, and physical trainers, in place will eliminate the need for trial and error.
- **Food deprivation and restriction:** Diets that eliminate foods or entire food groups can lead to cravings or unhealthy rebound eating.
- **Metabolic adaptation:** Over time, the body adapts to lower caloric intake by reducing energy expenditure. Staying on a lower-calorie diet for too long can hamper the body's metabolism.

Even GLP-1 users can have difficulty maintaining weight loss. The STEP 1 study, involving nearly 2,000 adults and published in April 2022, found that individuals who discontinued semaglutide medications regained two-thirds of the weight they had lost within a year. Improvements in the participants' cardiovascular markers were also reversed. This phenomenon is known as "Ozempic rebound." The 2024 SURMOUNT-4 clinical trial focused on tirzepatide, a dual GLP-1 and GIP medication. In this trial, researchers studied hundreds of participants in a double-blind placebo study focused on weight regain after discontinuing the medication. They found that 89.5 percent of participants who received tirzepatide for an additional fifty-two weeks maintained at least 80 percent of their initial weight loss, compared to only 16.6 percent in the placebo group which received no medication.

While the likelihood of weight rebound is concerning in itself, it's not a "net neutral" reverse back to your baseline weight. In fact, you will likely be in worse shape than when you originally started—even if your weight reverts back to the same number. Here's why: If you lost weight rapidly, you most likely lost anywhere from a small to substantial amount of muscle mass too. When you regain weight, you don't usually gain it back in the same proportions. There's a good chance you gain back fat in place of the muscle that was lost. In short, you may return to your original weight, but with a less favorable body composition. And the next time you attempt to lose weight, it may be even more challenging.

It's important to note that discontinuing a GLP-1 medication, for whatever reason, puts you at risk for significant weight regain if the proper steps are not taken. Many users struggle to maintain their dietary and lifestyle changes after stopping the medication due to the sudden shifts in appetite and hunger signaling. If you do end up stopping the medication, don't fret. It's not impossible to maintain your weight loss. The next sections will equip you with the right tools to keep the weight off.

Discontinuing GLP-1 Medication

Whether by choice or circumstance, many people end up discontinuing GLP-1 medications for a period or altogether. While these medications are marketed for lifelong use, not everyone is interested in ongoing treatment or has the resources to continue it. The medication is expensive, and many people don't have insurance that covers it. Even patients with insurance that covers GLP-1 may find that when they reach a lower BMI, their insurance stops covering the medication.

It's important to weigh the benefits against the potential negative side effects of chronic use. It's also worth noting that, as of this writing, there are no studies examining the effects of long-term use over several years or decades. If you are living with chronic endocrine dysregulation, it may be appropriate for you to continue taking the medication on a long-term basis. However, if weight loss is your only goal, long-term use is likely not suitable.

You may find that the time spent on GLP-1, even just for a short period of time, can be beneficial for kickstarting your body and establishing new eating and lifestyle habits. Creating new habits and routines while on the medication is essential for maintaining them if you transition off. While you're taking the medication, you can train yourself to eat healthier, reduce portion sizes, increase your activity, and listen to your hunger cues. If you don't change your behavior, the medication can serve only as a temporary solution. Reverting back to your old habits means the weight will start to creep back on.

When discontinuing the medication, many users report a rapid shift in appetite, satiety hormones, and food cravings, especially if stopping abruptly. Other users report exacerbated side effects, such as nausea, dizziness, and vomiting after stopping doses. There have also been anecdotal reports of temporary withdrawal symptoms similar to those experienced when weaning off an addictive substance, such as persistent headaches. It takes time for the medication to build up in your body—the reason doses are gradually increased. Similarly, it also takes time for it to clear from your system. Some users report it can take up to several weeks for the effects of the medication to wear off.

If you plan on stopping the medication, talk to your healthcare professional about tapering the dose down gradually to minimize complications. A sudden cessation of the medication can result in dangerous blood sugar dysregulation, particularly if you're using it to manage diabetes. A study presented at the European Congress on Obesity highlighted that patients were more successful in maintaining weight loss after a gradual tapering process (over nine weeks) combined with diet and lifestyle coaching.

Adjusting Your Diet after GLP-1

Once you are no longer taking the medication, you may notice your appetite coming back with a vengeance. It had been unnaturally suppressed, so it's normal and okay to feel hunger pangs again. Take your time to gradually increase your caloric intake. It's not realistic to maintain the abnormally low caloric intake you experienced while on the medication. During this transition period, it can be especially helpful to track your calories using an app like MyFitnessPal to ensure you make a healthy adjustment. If you were eating below your target caloric deficit, make it a goal to work your way back to that or stay there.

One way to deal with your returning hunger is to choose foods that provide more "bang for your buck" in terms of calories and volume. This approach, often called volume eating, focuses on low-calorie, nutrient-dense foods that help keep you feeling full. For example, 1 cup of pretzels has 150 calories, while 5 cups of popcorn also contain 150 calories. Similarly, 2 tablespoons of almonds have 100 calories, but so do 7 cups of celery. When you were on the medication, you were typically looking for high-calorie, high-nutrient foods. Now, you are aiming for low-calorie and nutrient-dense foods.

ESSENTIAL

The core concept of volume eating involves choosing foods that have a high water or fiber content. The idea is to fill up on foods that take up space in the stomach but are low in calories. Examples of low-calorie, high-volume foods include watermelon, leafy greens, cucumber, celery, apples, broth, popcorn, oats, and pickles.

As much as you can, stick to many of the same eating principles that you followed while taking the medication. Choose foods that are high in protein and fiber and contain moderate amounts of carbohydrates and fats. You don't necessarily have to go back to three large, traditional meals a day.

Sticking to smaller, more frequent meals can still be helpful for portion control and blood sugar management. Feel free to return to nutritious foods that you couldn't tolerate previously, like spicy foods and cruciferous vegetables, but continue to avoid or minimize processed and greasy, fried foods, as this will help you maintain a calorie deficit. If you do better following specific guidelines, a Mediterranean style of eating is a good starting point.

The Mediterranean diet emphasizes whole, minimally processed foods, healthy fats, and an active lifestyle. Studies have shown that it can lower blood pressure, improve cholesterol levels, stabilize blood sugar, and reduce the risk of cognitive decline. Here's a breakdown of its main components:

- Eat a wide variety of fruits and vegetables every day.
- Choose whole grains like barley, farro, brown rice, and whole-wheat products.
- Add healthy fats from nuts, seeds, and avocados to your diet. Replace butter and margarine with olive oil.
- Focus on fish, poultry, beans, and legumes. Red meat should be consumed rarely and in small amounts.
- Keep consumption of dairy products like yogurt and cheese to moderate amounts.
- Flavor meals with fresh herbs and spices instead of salt.
- Limit processed foods, refined sugars, and highly processed snacks to very rare occasions.
- Enjoy red wine in moderation (typically one glass per day for women, up to two for men), though it's not essential.

The antioxidants found in fruits, vegetables, olive oil, and nuts can also mimic the anti-inflammatory effects of the medication.

In addition to eating high-quality, nutrient-dense foods, keep up with the healthy habits that GLP-1 medication supported. Here are more tips to help you preserve your progress and minimize the chances of regaining weight:

- Make sure to drink water throughout the day—more water than you think you need. Dehydration can often be mistaken for hunger.
- Keep your meal timing consistent. Maintain regular intervals between eating to avoid extreme hunger, which can cause you to overeat. Try not to skip meals. This may lead to eating a larger meal later in the day.
- Continue to prioritize physical activity and strength training. Include a combination of aerobic exercises (like walking or cycling) and resistance training (using weights or body weight exercises) each week. This will help build lean muscle, which in turn boosts your metabolism.
- Manage your stress level and get enough sleep. Aim for 7–8 hours of sleep per night and find regular ways to manage stress, like meditation, yoga, or a calming bedtime routine.
- Be aware of emotional eating. Try to learn the difference between true hunger and emotional cravings. Learn ways to distract yourself from emotional cues.
- Check in with your healthcare providers. Regular check-ins with your doctor or nutritionist can help catch early signs of weight gain or metabolic changes. They can provide support and help you to adjust your approach.

Make sure you check in with yourself as well. If you notice that you're gradually gaining weight, re-evaluate your diet, exercise routine, and daily habits. Small adjustments can prevent substantial weight regain.

It will take time to readjust to your body's natural hunger and satiety cues. Coming off of the medication is a great opportunity to take up the practice of mindful eating. Mindful eating involves being fully present and engaged while eating, allowing you to honor your body's natural signals. Here are some core tenets of mindful eating:

- **Check in with yourself before eating.** Assess your physical and emotional state and consider if you are actually hungry.
- **Slow down your eating.** Take your time to enjoy each bite and reduce the pace of your eating.

- **Eat without distractions.** Minimize interruptions from screens or other activities to focus on your meal.
- **Savor your food.** Pay attention to the flavors, textures, and aromas of what you are eating.
- **Honor hunger and fullness cues.** Listen to your body to determine when you are hungry and when you are satisfied.

Practicing these principles facilitates a healthier relationship with food after GLP-1 medication. If you are tracking your calories, consider using an app that also incorporates hunger scales or encourages journaling emotions before and after eating, such as MyFitnessPal, Lose It!, or Cronometer.

ESSENTIAL

If you want to keep tight control on your blood sugar levels after GLP-1, talk to your physician about using a glucometer or continuous glucose monitor (CGM) for daily tracking. If your insurance doesn't cover a CGM, there are a new wave of companies, such as Nutrisense and Levels, who offer out-of-pocket payment for the monitors. For more data, consider a DEXA scan to evaluate your current body composition or an RMR (resting metabolic rate) test to measure the speed of your metabolism. These tests are often offered at local gyms or clinics and can provide helpful data as you navigate weight loss without GLP-1.

If you're looking for alternatives to mimic the effects of your GLP-1 medication, there are several well-researched supplements that may produce similar effects, though not as strongly or effectively as the medication itself:

- **Psyllium husk:** A soluble fiber found in food or supplement form that can boost GLP-1 levels
- **Berberine:** A plant-based compound that increases GLP-1 secretion through bitter taste receptors

- **Yerba maté:** A plant, often steeped to make tea, that increases GLP-1 production
- **Curcumin:** A compound found in turmeric that increases GLP-1 release

There are also a host of novel proprietary supplements, labeled as GLP-1 "boosters" or "activators," that are marketed as natural alternatives to the drug. So far, there isn't much research supporting these alternative products.

The Future of GLP-1 Weight Loss Medications

The research on GLP-1 and weight loss medications is still in its early stages. Many researchers didn't expect the medication to be as effective as it is, and many more are still trying to fully comprehend how it works in the first place. Is it working on the dopamine pathways? Is it working on the satiety system? What are the long-term implications of taking the medication? There are more questions than answers at the moment.

Lower-Dose Treatments

Currently, one of the biggest concerns about the medication is its unfavorable side effects. These effects can be so severe that some people stop using the medication altogether, while others force themselves to push through the discomfort. As the medication evolves, researchers are studying lower-dose treatment options that can be used long-term with fewer side effects—and also lower costs. Low-dose treatments could also potentially be used for weight maintenance or curbing unhealthy eating behaviors.

This idea of low-dose treatments, also known as microdosing, is gaining traction within various clinical specialties looking to use GLP-1 for disease treatment without the weight loss effects. For example, researchers are exploring the potential of GLP-1 for treating gut diseases like ulcerative colitis and Crohn's, as well as Alzheimer's, Parkinson's, dementia, and kidney disease. GLP-1's potential for treating all of these conditions lies in its ability to tame inflammation. Its range of uses may be much broader than originally anticipated.

Semaglutide, Tirzepatide, and Other Variations

As of the time of writing in 2024, semaglutide (Ozempic, Wegovy) and tirzepatide (Mounjaro, Zepbound) are the predominant GLP-1 agonists on the market. Novo Nordisk, the manufacturer of Ozempic, has a patent on semaglutide until at least 2031 in the United States. Due to this patent, the manufacturer has control over the production and pricing of the medication in the US. However, other countries have a much shorter patent timeline. The patent in Canada expires in 2026, and Sandoz Group AG is already planning to launch a generic version of semaglutide then.

The patent in China will also expire in 2026. Chinese developers have already been working on generic versions of Ozempic, and the patent was challenged in 2021 by a Chinese pharmaceutical company. Even though the patent was eventually upheld, they have still been developing their generic in anticipation of 2026.

In addition to semaglutide and tirzepatide, a new GLP-1 medication will soon hit the market. Eli Lilly, the manufacturer of Zepbound and Mounjaro, is currently developing a novel hormone receptor agonist with the active ingredient named retatrutide. It binds to the receptors of three hormones: glucose-dependent insulinotropic polypeptide (GIP), glucagon-like peptide-1 (GLP-1), and glucagon. A clinical trial showed that patients taking a weekly 8mg dose of retatrutide had an average body weight loss of 22.8 percent and those with a weekly 12mg dose had an average body weight loss of 24.2 percent. These trials seem to indicate that retatrutide is, so far, demonstrating more effective weight loss than semaglutide and tirzepatide. Eli Lilly researchers are still in phase 3 of clinical trials to get FDA approval, and the company hopes to have a product on the market soon.

QUESTION

What are generic and biosimilar medications?

A patent protects a company's exclusive right to manufacture a drug for a specific period. After a patent expires, companies can produce generic medications that are proven to be exact copies of synthetically made branded drugs. Biosimilars, on the other hand, closely resemble their target product but are derived from modified living organisms, such as yeast. Both generic and biosimilar versions of semaglutide are in the works.

Oral Medication Options

Due to the large size of the semaglutide molecule and challenges with gut absorption, developing effective oral medications has been difficult. To achieve a 1 percent absorption rate in the gut—necessary for an effective clinical dose—the oral dose must be 100 times stronger than the injectable form. Pharmaceutical companies are scrambling to find a solution.

Novo Nordisk, the manufacturer of Ozempic and Wegovy, is closing in on a new oral version of semaglutide for weight loss. They have already released an oral semaglutide for diabetes called Rybelsus, which is currently comparable in effectiveness to the lowest dose of the semaglutide injection. Their new weight loss drug, Amycretin, acts on GLP-1 and stimulates receptors for the amylin hormone, which regulates hunger. In trials, patients taking this oral medication lost up to 13 percent of their body weight over twelve weeks. It is still in phase 1 of clinical trials, so there is no timeline on when this drug may be on the market.

Pfizer and Eli Lilly are each developing their own small-molecule pill versions that would be less expensive than injections. Since the medication's initial safety has been established, research is expected to progress more rapidly thanks to a greater number of willing clinical participants and increased availability of funding.

GLP-1s and Substance Abuse

One of the most intriguing areas of emerging research is the use of GLP-1 for substance abuse treatment. Currently, the pharmaceutical options for opioid treatment are limited in comparison to how widespread opioid abuse is. Early phases of animal studies using GLP-1 show promising results. Elisabet Jerlhag, a researcher at the University of Gothenburg in Sweden, has noted that rats decrease their alcohol intake about 50 percent when injected with GLP-1 agonists. The same applies to other substances, such as cocaine, fentanyl, and heroin, which don't contribute any calories—indicating that GLP-1 has effects beyond just caloric regulation. The rats showed a significant decrease in dopamine levels and reduced cravings for the substances.

While this drop in dopamine can help diminish unwanted or unhealthy addictions, dopamine also plays a crucial role in fostering healthy habits, such as exercise, socialization, and the pursuit of personal goals, as well as more subtle behaviors like empathy. This aligns with reports from some users who found that the medication exacerbated their anxiety and depression, or decreased their overall motivation, likely due to the reduction in dopamine. Further research is needed to explore how to use the medication to treat addictions or unhealthy habits without compromising overall mental health.

What Else Can GLP-1s Do?

No one predicted the widespread success of GLP-1 medications. After previous attempts with medications mimicking other hormones like leptin and ghrelin failed, this medication was not expected to become the superstar it is today. Studies in rats and other animals, which didn't translate well into real-world efficacy, couldn't have predicted it either. Most scientists agree that the success of the drug was not because they fully understood the GLP-1 hormone, but rather because of luck. Appetite regulation is just the tip of the iceberg with GLP-1, as we venture into a new wave of treatments beyond obesity. The question has shifted from "What diseases can GLP-1 treat?" to "Which ones can't it help?" The world is eagerly watching and anticipating what this hormone will be able to achieve.

CHAPTER 5

Breakfast

Tomato and Mozzarella Baked Eggs

SERVES 6	
Calories	379g
Fat	26g
Sodium	560mg
Carbohydrates	15g
Fiber	3g
Sugar	8g
Protein	24g

This low-carb recipe is perfect for breakfast or even a quick dinner. Use full-fat mozzarella for optimal blood sugar regulation.

2 tablespoons unsalted butter

2 medium shallots, peeled and chopped

6 cloves garlic, peeled and minced

3 medium orange or yellow bell peppers, seeded and chopped

1 cup chopped white mushrooms

1 (14.5-ounce) can diced tomatoes, lightly drained

2 tablespoons fresh oregano leaves

1½ tablespoons chopped fresh rosemary

¼ cup chopped fresh basil

1 teaspoon chili powder

1 cup whole milk ricotta cheese

6 large eggs, room temperature

1 cup shredded Parmesan cheese

4 ounces fresh mozzarella cheese, diced

1 Heat butter in a large cast iron skillet over medium-high heat. Add shallots, garlic, peppers, and mushrooms. Cook until softened and almost caramelized, about 6–8 minutes.

2 Stir in tomatoes, oregano, rosemary, basil, and chili powder. Reduce heat to medium-low and cook for another 10 minutes, or until the mixture starts to thicken.

3 Preheat oven to 400°F.

4 Place six dollops of ricotta cheese over the tomato mixture. With a large spoon, create a well in each mound of ricotta. Crack an egg over each, careful not to let it run into the tomato mixture. Sprinkle with cheeses.

5 Bake for about 15 minutes (yolks will be slightly runny). Serve immediately.

Garlicky Veggie–Packed Omelet

Start your day off right with this nutrient-dense, low-carb omelet! Garlic is a versatile ingredient that has been shown to reduce blood sugar and cholesterol, so be generous with that ingredient!

2 teaspoons olive oil

1/4 cup chopped red onion

1/4 cup sliced button or cremini mushrooms

2 tablespoons water

1/2 cup torn fresh spinach leaves

1/4 cup chopped tomato

1/2 teaspoon garlic powder

2 large eggs

4 large egg whites

SERVES 2	
Calories	265
Fat	20g
Sodium	212mg
Carbohydrates	2g
Fiber	1g
Sugar	1g
Protein	19g

1 Heat oil in a medium skillet over medium heat.

2 Sauté onion for 1 minute. Add mushrooms and water, and sauté until mushrooms are softened, about 3–4 minutes.

3 Stir in spinach, tomato, and garlic powder and sauté for 2 minutes.

4 Whisk together eggs and egg whites in a medium bowl and pour over sautéed vegetables.

5 Immediately begin pushing the outer edges into the center with a spatula for one turn around the whole pan. Let omelet set for 2 minutes.

6 Gently slide the spatula under omelet and quickly flip. Continue cooking omelet for another 3–5 minutes, or until no longer runny. Slide onto a plate, folding into thirds as the omelet comes out of skillet. Cut omelet in half and serve warm.

Tempeh, Tomato, and Spinach Omelet

SERVES 2	
Calories	247
Fat	14g
Sodium	618mg
Carbohydrates	10g
Fiber	4g
Sugar	3g
Protein	20g

WHAT IS TEMPEH?

Tempeh is an Indonesian food made from soybeans. While tofu and tempeh are similar, tofu is made from soy curds and tempeh is made from fermented whole soybeans. It has a chewier, crumbly texture and a nutty flavor. It's packed with fiber, probiotics, and tons of plant-based protein.

Say hello to tempeh, the high-protein cousin of tofu! Tomatoes, spinach, and tempeh are all low-glycemic ingredients, which can curb your blood sugar levels.

2 large eggs

3 large egg whites

¼ teaspoon salt

1 (10-ounce) package frozen chopped spinach, thawed and squeezed dry

1 cup chopped tomato

¼ cup cooked julienned tempeh

1 tablespoon olive oil

1 Beat eggs and egg whites in a small bowl. Mix in salt.
2 Place spinach in a medium microwavable bowl. Microwave on high for about 2 minutes or until warm and soft. Stir in tomato and tempeh.
3 Heat oil in a medium skillet over low heat. Pour egg mixture into the pan. Cook until edges show firmness, about 2 minutes. Add spinach mixture evenly over eggs. Fold one side over the other and cook for 1 minute. Flip omelet and cook for 30 seconds more. Transfer to a plate. Cut omelet in half and serve.

Veggie Egg Beater Omelet

If you're struggling to consume full meals, this simple, five-ingredient omelet is a lighter option that may be easier to tolerate in the morning. To increase the protein, add more Egg Beaters.

SERVES 2	
Calories	160
Fat	7g
Sodium	219mg
Carbohydrates	9g
Fiber	2g
Sugar	4g
Protein	15g

1 cup Egg Beaters Liquid Egg Substitute

½ cup water

1 cup chopped tomato

1 cup chopped green or yellow bell pepper

1 tablespoon olive oil

1 Beat Egg Beaters with water in a small bowl. Mix tomato and pepper in another small bowl.

2 Heat olive oil in a small skillet over low heat. Pour Egg Beater mixture into the pan. Cook until edges show firmness, about 2 minutes. Add vegetable mixture evenly over eggs. Fold one side over the other and cook for 1 minute. Flip omelet and cook for 30 seconds more. Transfer to a plate, cut in half, and serve.

Chili Masala Tofu Scramble

This vegan and gluten-free breakfast will satisfy your spice cravings. Both cumin and turmeric boast anti-inflammatory benefits.

SERVES 2	
Calories	290
Fat	18g
Sodium	109mg
Carbohydrates	14g
Fiber	3g
Sugar	6g
Protein	18g

2 tablespoons olive oil

1 yellow onion, peeled and diced

2 cloves garlic, peeled and minced

1 (14-ounce) package firm or extra-firm tofu, drained, pressed, and cut into 1" cubes

1 medium green bell pepper, seeded and chopped

¾ cup sliced button mushrooms

1 tablespoon low-sodium soy sauce

1 teaspoon curry powder

½ teaspoon ground cumin

¼ teaspoon ground turmeric

1 teaspoon nutritional yeast

1 In a large skillet, heat oil over medium-high heat. Add onion and garlic and sauté for 4–5 minutes until soft.

2 Stir in tofu, pepper, mushrooms, soy sauce, curry powder, cumin, and turmeric. Sauté for 6–8 minutes until tofu is lightly browned.

3 Remove from heat and stir in nutritional yeast. Serve immediately.

Baked "Sausage" and Mushroom Frittata

This high-protein frittata will help you maintain healthy muscle mass. Both tofu and nutritional yeast are excellent sources of protein for vegans or people who want to reduce the amount of animal products in their diet.

SERVES 4	
Calories	333
Fat	17g
Sodium	622mg
Carbohydrates	9g
Fiber	1g
Sugar	2g
Protein	36g

VEGAN "MEAT"

Vegan meat, sometimes called plant-based meat, is a meat substitute made with soy, peas, fava beans, mushrooms, or other vegan ingredients. Plant-based meat is an excellent addition to your diet because it's lower in saturated fat, which can exacerbate gastrointestinal symptoms, than animal meat. It's also higher in fiber, which helps regulate your blood sugar.

2 tablespoons olive oil

1/2 large yellow onion, peeled and diced

3 cloves garlic, peeled and minced

1/2 cup sliced white mushrooms

1 (12-ounce) package vegan sausage or vegan beef crumbles

3/4 teaspoon salt

1/4 teaspoon ground black pepper

1 (14-ounce) package firm tofu, drained and pressed

1 (14-ounce) package silken tofu, drained

1 tablespoon soy sauce

2 tablespoons nutritional yeast

1/4 teaspoon ground turmeric

1 medium tomato, thinly sliced

1 Preheat oven to 325°F. Spray a 9" glass pie dish with nonstick cooking spray.

2 In a large skillet, heat oil over medium heat. Add onion, garlic, mushrooms, and vegan sausage. Sauté for 3–4 minutes until sausage is browned and mushrooms are soft. Transfer to a large bowl. Season with salt and pepper and set aside.

3 Add firm tofu, silken tofu, soy sauce, nutritional yeast, and turmeric to a blender. Process until smooth. Add to sausage mixture and stir to combine. Pour into prepared dish. Top with tomato slices.

4 Bake for 40–45 minutes until firm. Cool for 5–10 minutes before serving.

Mediterranean Frittata

You'll love this hearty frittata that can be enjoyed throughout the week or frozen for later. Freeze additional portions in a freezer-safe container for up to two months.

1 pound Idaho potatoes, sliced

3 large red bell peppers, seeded and sliced

1 large yellow onion, peeled and sliced

2 teaspoons olive oil

1/2 teaspoon coarse salt

1/4 teaspoon cracked black pepper

3 large eggs

6 large egg whites

1 cup plain low-fat Greek yogurt

1 cup whole milk

3 ounces fontina cheese, grated

1/2 bunch fresh oregano, chopped

1 Preheat oven to 375°F.
2 In a large bowl, toss potatoes, bell peppers, and onion and spread out in a large ungreased roasting pan. Season with salt and black pepper. Roast vegetables for 20–25 minutes until partially cooked.
3 Transfer vegetables to an ungreased 9" × 13" baking dish.
4 Whisk together eggs, egg whites, yogurt, milk, and cheese in a medium bowl. Pour egg mixture over vegetables in the baking dish. Bake until egg mixture is completely set, approximately 30–35 minutes. Sprinkle with oregano and serve.

SERVES 6	
Calories	304
Fat	15g
Sodium	226mg
Carbohydrates	22g
Fiber	3g
Sugar	7g
Protein	20g

OREGANO AND BLOOD SUGAR

According to recent studies, compounds in oregano may help to improve insulin resistance and reduce blood sugar levels by inhibiting cravings for sweets. Oregano also has antioxidant, anti-inflammatory, and antifungal properties, making it a great addition to your diet while enhancing your meals with fresh flavors!

Huevos Rancheros Breakfast Casserole

The extra egg whites in this comforting casserole provide an extra dose of protein. Fiber-rich black beans help to keep the GI tract running smoothly.

SERVES 6	
Calories	384
Fat	20g
Sodium	804mg
Carbohydrates	25g
Fiber	8g
Sugar	5g
Protein	26g

BENEFITS OF DIETARY FIBER

Fiber refers to the part of the plant that our bodies can't break down. Fiber is important for a healthy digestive system, and it supports overall gastrointestinal health. Fiber can help you feel full longer, and because it isn't absorbed well, it doesn't contribute to blood sugar level spikes. Dietary fiber is also linked to other benefits, such as hormone balance, cancer prevention, and a reduced risk of gallstones and kidney stones.

1 tablespoon vegetable oil

1 large yellow onion, peeled and chopped

1 medium green bell pepper, seeded and chopped

1 (15-ounce) can black beans, drained and rinsed

1/2 cup salsa

6 large eggs

6 large egg whites

1 cup nonfat milk

3 tablespoons chopped fresh cilantro

1/2 teaspoon salt

1/2 cup shredded extra-sharp Cheddar cheese

1 Preheat oven to 375°F and lightly spray a 9" × 13" casserole dish with nonstick cooking spray.

2 Heat oil over medium-high heat in a large nonstick skillet. Sauté onion and pepper until softened, about 5 minutes. Spread vegetable mixture on the bottom of the casserole dish in an even layer. Spread beans, then salsa, over vegetables.

3 Whisk eggs, egg whites, milk, cilantro, and salt together in a large bowl. Pour over casserole dish, then sprinkle cheese on top.

4 Bake casserole, uncovered, on the middle rack until it is set in the center, 45–50 minutes. Serve warm.

Spinach and Pasta Frittata

Pasta for breakfast—what a treat! Try swapping out the regular spaghetti with a pasta made with chickpeas or lentils. They have four times as much fiber and twice the protein as flour-based pasta. Legumes are also a great source of iron.

½ pound spaghetti, cooked according to package directions

½ cup finely diced fontina cheese

½ cup grated Parmesan cheese

1 (10-ounce) package frozen chopped spinach, thawed and squeezed dry

2 tablespoons chopped fresh parsley

3 large eggs, lightly beaten

½ teaspoon salt

½ teaspoon ground black pepper

1 tablespoon unsalted butter

1. In a large bowl, mix together spaghetti, cheeses, spinach, parsley, eggs, salt, and pepper.
2. Melt butter in a very large nonstick skillet over medium heat. Add the pasta mixture and spread evenly over the pan. Cook for 5–6 minutes until the bottom is set. Invert the frittata onto a large plate, then slip it back into the skillet and cook until completely set, about 3 minutes.
3. Cut into wedges and serve.

SERVES 4	
Calories	300
Fat	16g
Sodium	883mg
Carbohydrates	21g
Fiber	3g
Sugar	1g
Protein	18g

SUPER SPINACH

Not only is spinach high in fiber but it also contains a special antioxidant called alpha-lipoic acid that has been shown to increase insulin sensitivity, prevent oxidative stress, and even relieve symptoms of neuropathy, a nerve disorder commonly caused by diabetes that can cause pain, numbness, tingling, and weakness in the hands, feet, or other parts of the body.

Mexican Egg Brunch

SERVES 4

Calories	393
Fat	25g
Sodium	414mg
Carbohydrates	19g
Fiber	4g
Sugar	4g
Protein	23g

If you like migas, a Tex-Mex favorite breakfast of scrambled eggs, corn tortillas, onions, and peppers, you'll love this easy casserole version. It's gluten-free, high in protein, and delicious!

2 cups corn tortilla chips

1 cup shredded Cheddar cheese, divided

4 large eggs

4 large egg whites

1 medium red bell pepper, seeded and chopped

1 medium jalapeño pepper, seeded and chopped (optional)

2 cups halved cherry tomatoes

½ medium avocado, peeled, pitted, and chopped

¼ cup chopped fresh cilantro

1 Preheat oven to 400°F. Grease a 9" × 13" glass casserole dish.

2 Spread tortilla chips in casserole dish. Top with ½ cup cheese.

3 In a medium bowl, whisk eggs and egg whites until fluffy. Pour eggs into casserole dish. Sprinkle on remaining ½ cup cheese. Top with bell pepper and jalapeño.

4 Bake for 15 minutes or until eggs are firm around edges of the casserole dish.

5 Top with tomatoes, avocado, and cilantro before serving.

"Sausage" Egg Cups

If you're a fan of Starbucks's egg bites, this copycat recipe will be a winner for you! Once you get comfortable with the recipe, play around with your favorite ground meat and vegetable combinations. Try ground beef, pork, or chicken and mushrooms, bell peppers, or tomatoes.

SERVES 6	
Calories	265
Fat	17g
Sodium	365mg
Carbohydrates	4g
Fiber	2g
Sugar	1g
Protein	24g

1/2 **pound ground turkey**

1/2 **teaspoon dried sage**

1/2 **teaspoon salt**

1/2 **teaspoon ground black pepper**

1/4 **medium yellow onion, peeled and chopped**

1/4 **cup chopped zucchini**

12 **large eggs**

1 **large avocado, peeled, pitted, and diced**

1 Preheat oven to 350°F. Grease a 12-cup muffin pan with a small amount of coconut oil.

2 Heat a large skillet over medium heat and add ground turkey, sage, salt, and pepper. Cook, stirring, until turkey is no longer pink, about 5 minutes. Remove turkey mixture with a slotted spoon and set aside in a medium bowl. Add onion and zucchini to pan and sauté until tender, about 4 minutes. Add cooked onion and zucchini to turkey mixture.

3 Add eggs to bowl and stir until combined. Pour mixture evenly into the prepared muffin pan.

4 Bake for 30 minutes or until egg is cooked through.

5 Top each egg cup with a few pieces of avocado. Serve warm or at room temperature.

Chocolate Peanut Butter Smoothie

SERVES 2	
Calories	216
Fat	11g
Sodium	126mg
Carbohydrates	16g
Fiber	4g
Sugar	9g
Protein	14g

AN EASY SMOOTHIE FORMULA

Smoothies are great for those days when you don't have the appetite for a full meal but still want to get your calories in. Use this formula for a balanced smoothie: 1 cup liquid base (any type of milk or water), a source of fiber (1 tablespoon flaxseed or psyllium husk), some protein (try 1 tablespoon nut butter or 1 scoop of protein powder), and ½ cup chopped fruits and/ or vegetables.

If you're having trouble consuming enough calories, keep this recipe on hand! Peanut butter is high in calories without being too filling. Feel free to go over the serving size if you are able to tolerate it.

2 tablespoons unsweetened cocoa powder

2 tablespoons natural creamy peanut butter

½ medium banana, peeled, sliced, and frozen

½ cup Fairlife Whole Ultra-Filtered Milk

½ cup plain low-fat Greek yogurt

½ teaspoon vanilla extract

4 ice cubes

Combine all ingredients in a blender and blend until thick and creamy. Serve immediately.

Coffee and Chocolate Yogurt Parfaits

Who turns down chocolate for breakfast? This parfait is a great option when you want to eat something sweet without raising your blood sugar levels too much. The pumpkin seeds, chia seeds, and almonds are high in fiber and protein, which stabilize blood sugar spikes.

¼ cup shelled raw pumpkin seeds

½ cup chopped almonds

¼ cup semisweet chocolate chips

2 tablespoons chia seeds

1 tablespoon ground flaxseed

¼ teaspoon salt

24 ounces plain low-fat Greek yogurt

½ tablespoon instant espresso powder

¼ cup maple syrup

1 In a medium bowl, combine pumpkin seeds, almonds, chocolate chips, chia seeds, flaxseed, and salt. In another bowl, whisk together yogurt, espresso powder, and maple syrup.

2 To assemble parfaits, spoon ¼ cup yogurt mixture into four (8-ounce) sealable jars.

3 Top yogurt with 2 tablespoons nut and seed mixture. Repeat layers until all ingredients have been used. Seal jars and store in the refrigerator for up to four days.

SERVES 4	
Calories	433
Fat	23g
Sodium	211mg
Carbohydrates	33g
Fiber	6g
Sugar	25g
Protein	24g

SEEDS—SUPERFOODS WITH SUPER FIBER

Chia seeds have some of the highest fiber content out there, even more than nuts, beans, and other grains. In fact, 1 ounce of chia seeds (about 2 tablespoons) provides 9.75 grams of fiber. Other seeds are good sources of fiber as well, including flaxseeds (8 grams per ounce). Hemp seeds contain 1 gram of fiber per ounce, but they provide 10 grams of protein.

Cinnamon Smoothie

SERVES 2	
Calories	166
Fat	4g
Sodium	93mg
Carbohydrates	25g
Fiber	2g
Sugar	14g
Protein	8g

Adding oatmeal to smoothies is a great way to sneak in a bit of extra fiber. The trick is to grind the oats into a powder before adding it to the smoothie. You can do this in a high-powdered blender, coffee grinder, or food processor. Powdered oats combined with a frozen banana create a thick, satisfying smoothie.

¼ cup rolled oats, ground into a powder

1 cup unsweetened almond milk

½ cup plain low-fat Greek yogurt

1 medium banana, peeled, sliced, and frozen

1 teaspoon honey

1 teaspoon ground cinnamon

Combine all ingredients in a blender and blend until smooth, about 1 minute. Enjoy immediately.

Toast with Gorgonzola, Apple, and Honey

SERVES 4	
Calories	397
Fat	17g
Sodium	565mg
Carbohydrates	46g
Fiber	5g
Sugar	26g
Protein	17g

For an extra energy boost in the morning, try this sweet and savory toast recipe. Using whole-grain or sourdough bread helps to lower the glycemic index. To keep the carbohydrate count even lower, reduce the amount of honey.

4 (1-ounce) slices whole-grain bread, toasted

8 ounces crumbled Gorgonzola cheese

1 medium Fuji apple, cored and thinly sliced

¼ cup honey

Spread each bread slice with 2 ounces Gorgonzola. Lay apple slices on top and drizzle honey over them. Serve immediately.

Overnight Maple Walnut N'Oatmeal

If you're short on time in the mornings, overnight oats need to be part of your breakfast rotation. This nutty porridge is a great source of protein and anti-inflammatory fats to keep you satisfied all morning.

2/3 cup Fairlife Whole Ultra-Filtered Milk

1/2 cup hemp hearts

1 tablespoon chia seeds

1 tablespoon maple syrup

1/2 teaspoon vanilla extract

1/8 teaspoon sea salt

2 tablespoons finely chopped walnuts

1 Combine all ingredients in a medium bowl and mix well.

2 Divide mixture in half and pour into two (8-ounce) wide-mouthed Mason jars. Cover and refrigerate overnight. Serve cold.

SERVES 2	
Calories	379
Fat	28g
Sodium	188mg
Carbohydrates	13g
Fiber	3g
Sugar	10g
Protein	19g

HEART-Y AND HEALTHY

Hemp hearts are the soft inner part of the hemp seed, known for their mild, nutty flavor. They are rich in omega-3 and omega-6 fatty acids that can help reduce the risk of heart disease. Hemp seeds contain all nine essential amino acids and are high in protein. Toss a nutritious spoonful into smoothies, oatmeal, salads, or your favorite baked treat.

Danish Egg Cake with Bacon and Tomatoes

SERVES 6	
Calories	207
Fat	12g
Sodium	478mg
Carbohydrates	8g
Fiber	1g
Sugar	4g
Protein	17g

This fluffy Scandinavian oven-baked pancake rises like a soufflé as it cooks. It's an ideal dish to share with a group for an indulgent brunch. Lean turkey bacon is easier to digest than regular bacon.

6 strips turkey bacon, cut into 1/2" pieces

1/3 cup minced yellow onion

2 cups diced tomatoes

8 large eggs

1/4 cup all-purpose flour

2 cups Fairlife Whole Ultra-Filtered Milk

1 teaspoon baking powder

1/4 teaspoon salt

1/8 teaspoon ground black pepper

1 tablespoon chopped fresh parsley

1 Preheat oven to 425°F.

2 In a large oven-proof skillet over medium heat, fry bacon until crisp, stirring occasionally to prevent burning. Transfer bacon to a paper towel–covered plate. Discard all but 1 teaspoon of bacon fat from the pan. Use a pastry brush to grease the bottom and sides of the pan with the remaining fat.

3 In a medium bowl, toss bacon with onion and tomatoes. Set aside.

4 In a large bowl, whisk together eggs, flour, milk, baking powder, salt, and pepper and pour into the skillet. Cook over medium-high heat for 2 minutes, then transfer to the oven.

5 Bake for 15 minutes, or until puffed and golden. Remove from oven and spoon bacon-tomato mixture in the middle of pancake. Sprinkle with parsley, cut into wedges, and serve immediately.

High-Protein Cottage Cheese Pancakes

Cottage cheese is a smart choice for breakfast because it's high in protein and low in carbohydrates. And it makes delicious pancakes!

1 cup low-fat cottage cheese

3 large eggs

2 tablespoons butter

¼ cup all-purpose flour

1 teaspoon vanilla extract

¼ teaspoon salt

1 Drain liquid from cottage cheese by placing it in a strainer for 1 hour.

2 Place drained cottage cheese, eggs, butter, flour, vanilla, and salt in a mixing bowl. Beat until well blended. Cover and let stand for 30 minutes.

3 Spray a large skillet with nonstick cooking spray and heat over medium-low heat. Cook pancakes for 4–5 minutes, turning once, until golden brown. Serve hot.

SERVES 3	
Calories	232
Fat	15g
Sodium	549mg
Carbohydrates	9g
Fiber	0g
Sugar	3g
Protein	15g

WHIPPED COTTAGE CHEESE

If you aren't a fan of the texture of cottage cheese, don't fret! Blend your cottage cheese in a blender or food processor for 30–60 seconds until you achieve a smooth, creamy texture. Add milk if you want a silkier consistency. Whipping cottage cheese creates a texture that's perfect for dips, spreads, or adding to smoothies.

Perfect Poached Eggs on Toast

SERVES 1	
Calories	319
Fat	14g
Sodium	203mg
Carbohydrates	27g
Fiber	4g
Sugar	12g
Protein	21g

Poaching an egg is a great way to enjoy this nutrient-dense food. It's not hard to do once you get the hang of it. Poached eggs are wonderful on toast, but you can also try a lighter version with tomato slices instead.

2 teaspoons apple cider vinegar

1 teaspoon salt

2 extra-large eggs

2 (1-ounce) slices whole-wheat bread, toasted

1/8 teaspoon ground black pepper

1 Place a 2-quart saucepan filled with 2" of water over medium heat. Add vinegar and salt and bring to a simmer (don't allow water to boil).

2 Meanwhile, break eggs into ramekins or coffee cups.

3 When the water is simmering, use a spoon to stir it in one direction until the water is swirling around. Carefully drop the eggs, one at a time, into the center of the "whirlpool." This helps keep the eggs together in the water. You can use a spatula to help it along if you need to.

4 Turn off the heat, and cover the pan for exactly 5 minutes. Do not lift the lid. Have a slotted spoon ready to retrieve the eggs when done. After 5 minutes, carefully lift eggs out with the slotted spoon and onto toast. Serve immediately with a sprinkle of pepper.

Shakshuka for Two

Shakshuka is a popular dish from the Middle East and North Africa that bursts with depth and flavor in every bite. Chickpeas are the star of the show in this version, providing a significant source of protein, fiber, and B vitamins.

SERVES 2	
Calories	443
Fat	27g
Sodium	926mg
Carbohydrates	28g
Fiber	8g
Sugar	12g
Protein	22g

1 tablespoon olive oil

1/2 cup canned chickpeas, drained and rinsed

1/2 large green bell pepper, seeded and diced

1/2 teaspoon smoked paprika

1/2 teaspoon ground cumin

1/4 teaspoon ground turmeric

1/16 teaspoon garlic powder

1/8 teaspoon salt

1/2 teaspoon ground black pepper

1 (14.5-ounce) can crushed tomatoes

1 tablespoon tomato paste

1 teaspoon light brown sugar

1/2 teaspoon rice wine vinegar

1/4 cup crumbled goat cheese

2 large eggs

1/2 cup crumbled feta cheese

2 tablespoons chopped fresh cilantro

1 Heat oil in a large, wide skillet over medium-high heat. Add chickpeas, bell pepper, paprika, cumin, turmeric, garlic powder, salt, and black pepper. Cook for 5 minutes, stirring occasionally.

2 Add tomatoes, tomato paste, sugar, and vinegar; reduce heat to medium and cook for 12–15 minutes until sauce is slightly thickened. Stir in goat cheese.

3 Remove skillet from heat. Make two wells in sauce and crack an egg into each indentation. Use a spatula to pull some of egg whites slightly out of wells, being careful not to touch yolks. Sprinkle feta over top.

4 Place skillet back on burner over medium-low heat. Gently simmer for 10 minutes. Cover and cook for 3–5 minutes until eggs are cooked to desired doneness. Top with cilantro. Serve hot.

Freezer Breakfast Burritos with Sautéed Vegetables

SERVES 8	
Calories	424
Fat	17g
Sodium	601mg
Carbohydrates	38g
Fiber	11g
Sugar	3g
Protein	30g

These savory burritos are bursting with protein! To cut down on prep time, use frozen pre-diced onions and bell peppers.

1 tablespoon olive oil

1 medium white onion, peeled and sliced

1 large red bell pepper, seeded and sliced

1 large yellow bell pepper, seeded and sliced

1 large orange bell pepper, seeded and sliced

12 large eggs

¼ cup whole milk

¼ teaspoon salt

⅛ teaspoon ground black pepper

2 tablespoons unsalted butter

8 (12") low-carb tortillas

1½ cups shredded Monterey jack cheese

2 cups baby spinach

2 (15-ounce) cans low-sodium black beans, drained and rinsed

1 Heat oil in a large skillet over medium-high heat. Sauté onion and bell peppers until tender and onion is translucent, about 12 minutes. Remove from heat and set aside.

2 In a large bowl, whisk together eggs, milk, salt, and black pepper until well combined.

3 In the same skillet over medium heat, melt butter. Add egg mixture and cook, stirring constantly, until mostly set but still moist, about 6 minutes. Remove from heat and let cool completely.

4 Place a tortilla on a 10" × 16" piece of aluminum foil. Sprinkle 3 tablespoons cheese onto the lower third of the tortilla. Top with ¼ cup spinach, 1½ tablespoons black beans, 3 tablespoons scrambled eggs, and ¼ cup pepper mixture. Roll the burrito tightly by folding the sides over the filling, then rolling from the bottom up. Wrap the burrito tightly in the aluminum foil.

5 Repeat with remaining ingredients. Freeze in a single layer on a baking sheet. Transfer frozen burritos to a gallon-sized zip-top plastic freezer bag. When ready to eat, heat in a 350°F oven for 20 minutes or unwrap burrito and microwave on high for 2 minutes.

CHAPTER 6

Poultry and Beef

Ginger Chicken Salad

This salad is filled with warming spices from the vinaigrette. The small amount of ginger can help to reduce nausea as well.

SERVES 4	
Calories	278
Fat	14g
Sodium	689mg
Carbohydrates	7g
Fiber	3g
Sugar	1g
Protein	31g

AN EASY SOURCE OF PROTEIN

A whole rotisserie chicken can provide you with several small meals' worth of protein with no cooking required. Top a salad with a few ounces, shred some dark meat and toss with a peanut sauce for lettuce wraps, or just nibble on a wing when you need a quick snack.

3 tablespoons olive oil

1 tablespoon rice wine vinegar

1 tablespoon lemon juice

1 tablespoon grated fresh ginger

2 teaspoons five-spice powder

$1/2$ teaspoon salt

$1/2$ teaspoon ground black pepper

8 cups chopped red leaf lettuce

3 cups shredded rotisserie chicken breast

4 small radishes, trimmed and sliced

2 scallions, trimmed and thinly sliced

2 tablespoons roughly chopped flat-leaf parsley

1 In a small bowl, whisk together oil, vinegar, lemon juice, ginger, five-spice powder, salt, and pepper.

2 In a large bowl, toss together lettuce, chicken, radishes, and scallions.

3 Drizzle the dressing over the salad and toss well to coat. Garnish with parsley before serving.

Slow Cooker Chicken and Vegetable Soup

Let your slow cooker do the heavy lifting! This is your easy, go-to light meal for the days you're feeling the side effects of GLP-1. You get a healthy dose of protein and nutrients while going easy on digestion.

2 stalks celery, finely diced

1 large sweet onion, peeled and diced

1 large yellow bell pepper, seeded and chopped

1 tablespoon olive oil

1 teaspoon butter, melted

1 clove garlic, peeled and minced

4 cups low-sodium chicken broth

6 medium potatoes, peeled and diced

1 bay leaf

1/4 teaspoon salt

1/8 teaspoon ground black pepper

4 (4-ounce) boneless, skinless chicken breasts, cut into bite-sized pieces

1 (10-ounce) package frozen green beans

1 (10-ounce) package frozen corn

1 (10-ounce) package frozen baby peas

2 teaspoons fresh parsley

1 Add celery, onion, bell pepper, oil, and butter to a 4–6-quart slow cooker. Stir to coat vegetables in oil and butter. Cover and cook on high for 30 minutes or until vegetables are soft.

2 Stir in garlic, broth, potatoes, bay leaf, salt, black pepper, and chicken. Cover and cook on low for 6 hours.

3 Remove and discard bay leaf. Stir in green beans, corn, and peas; cover and cook on low for 1 hour or until vegetables are heated through. Top with parsley before serving.

SERVES 8	
Calories	315
Fat	6g
Sodium	259mg
Carbohydrates	39g
Fiber	7g
Sugar	7g
Protein	26g

THAWING FROZEN VEGETABLES

There are several safe ways to thaw frozen vegetables, but they should never be left out at room temperature. One option is to place them in the refrigerator until fully defrosted. Another method is to use the defrost setting on your microwave, stirring every 60 seconds. Alternatively, you can skip the thawing altogether and cook them straight from frozen.

Instant Pot® Turmeric Chicken and Cabbage Soup

SERVES 6

Calories	254
Fat	13g
Sodium	371mg
Carbohydrates	11g
Fiber	2g
Sugar	4g
Protein	23g

THE GOLDEN SPICE

Turmeric comes from the root of a plant in the same family as ginger. Known for its bright orange color, turmeric's flavor is earthy and peppery, and it also has a lot of health benefits. The active ingredient of turmeric is curcumin, which has strong anti-inflammatory properties. Moreover, research indicates that turmeric may have cancer-fighting properties by inhibiting tumor growth.

This pressure cooker soup is a powerhouse meal with ingredients that combat inflammation, nausea, and blood sugar spikes all at once. Use the turmeric and ginger generously!

2 tablespoons olive oil

4 (4-ounce) boneless, skinless chicken thighs

½ teaspoon salt

½ teaspoon ground black pepper

3 tablespoons minced fresh ginger

3 large carrots, peeled and thinly sliced

1 large red onion, peeled and diced

2 teaspoons ground turmeric

8 cups low-sodium chicken broth

3 cups thinly sliced green cabbage

2 tablespoons chopped flat-leaf parsley

1 Press the Sauté button on an Instant Pot® and heat oil. Add chicken, season with salt and pepper, and brown for 3 minutes per side. Add ginger, carrots, and onion to the pot. Sauté for 5 minutes.

2 Stir in turmeric and broth and stir well to loosen any bits that are stuck to the bottom. Press the Cancel button. Close lid, press the Manual or Pressure Cook button, and adjust time to 12 minutes.

3 When the timer beeps, let pressure release naturally for 10 minutes, then quick-release remaining steam. Press the Cancel button, open lid, and stir well.

4 Stir in cabbage and press the Sauté button. Cook until cabbage has wilted, 5 minutes.

5 Ladle soup into individual bowls and garnish with parsley. Serve immediately.

Chicken and Vegetable Frittata

A frittata is an easy high-protein option for any meal. The addition of chicken breast makes this a hearty choice for lunch or dinner. To increase the protein even more, add a few egg whites to the mix.

1 teaspoon butter

3 small shallots, peeled and sliced

2 cloves garlic, peeled and minced

8 ounces boneless, skinless chicken breasts, diced

1/2 teaspoon salt

1/4 teaspoon ground black pepper

1 cup chopped zucchini

12 asparagus spears, trimmed and cut into 1" pieces

8 large eggs

1/2 cup 2% milk

1/4 cup grated Parmesan cheese

SERVES 4	
Calories	287
Fat	15g
Sodium	752mg
Carbohydrates	6g
Fiber	1g
Sugar	2g
Protein	32g

1 Preheat oven to 350°F. Spray a medium square or round casserole dish with nonstick cooking spray.

2 Melt butter in a large skillet over medium heat and sauté shallots and garlic until soft, about 3 minutes.

3 Add chicken and sprinkle with salt and pepper. Sauté until chicken is cooked, about 8 minutes. Stir in zucchini and asparagus and sauté 2 minutes or until vegetables are tender-crisp.

4 Pour chicken mixture into the prepared pan.

5 In a large bowl, whisk together eggs, milk, and Parmesan and pour over contents in the dish.

6 Bake for 20–25 minutes until eggs are set and just starting to brown. Serve hot or at room temperature.

WHAT'S A FRITTATA?

Omelets, frittatas, and quiche—what's the difference among them? A frittata is an Italian-style egg dish that resembles an omelet but is thicker and often baked. A quiche typically has a crust, while frittatas are crustless. In contrast, omelets are cooked quickly and usually folded around various fillings.

Chicken Mushroom Marinara Bake

SERVES 4	
Calories	461
Fat	16g
Sodium	923mg
Carbohydrates	43g
Fiber	7g
Sugar	8g
Protein	36g

Combine chicken, marinara sauce, and mushrooms with high-protein pasta for an easy dinner. To reduce the prep time even more, grab a rotisserie chicken from the grocery store.

2 tablespoons butter or olive oil

1 pound white mushrooms, sliced

1 (16-ounce) jar marinara sauce

1 cup cooked and diced chicken breast

8 ounces lentil or chickpea pasta, cooked according to package directions

1 teaspoon dried basil

1/2 teaspoon garlic salt

1 cup shredded mozzarella cheese

1 Preheat oven to 350°F. Grease a medium casserole dish; set aside.

2 Heat butter or oil in a large skillet over medium heat. Add mushrooms and sauté for 5 minutes or until tender. Transfer to a large bowl.

3 Add marinara sauce, chicken, and cooked pasta to the bowl and stir to combine. Pour into prepared casserole dish. Sprinkle basil and garlic salt evenly over casserole. Top with cheese.

4 Bake for 30 minutes or until cheese is slightly browned and sauce is bubbly. Allow to cool for 5 minutes before serving.

Chicken and Bean Tacos

Get a double dose of protein with this quick, flavorful 15-minute taco recipe. Use a mild salsa to decrease any digestive stress.

1 pound boneless, skinless chicken breasts, cut into 1" cubes

1/2 teaspoon salt

1/8 teaspoon ground black pepper

1 tablespoon arrowroot powder

2 tablespoons olive oil

1 large yellow onion, peeled and chopped

1 medium yellow bell pepper, seeded and chopped

1 (15-ounce) can Great Northern beans, drained and rinsed

1 cup salsa

8 corn taco shells

2 cups shredded iceberg lettuce

1 cup halved grape tomatoes

1/2 cup sour cream

1 cup shredded Cheddar cheese

SERVES 8	
Calories	343
Fat	17g
Sodium	797mg
Carbohydrates	21g
Fiber	5g
Sugar	4g
Protein	26g

1 Heat oven to 350°F.

2 Sprinkle chicken with salt, black pepper, and arrowroot powder.

3 Heat oil in a large skillet over medium heat and add chicken. Cook and stir until almost cooked, about 4 minutes; remove from skillet. Add onion and bell pepper to skillet; cook and stir 4–5 minutes until crisp-tender.

4 Return chicken to skillet along with beans and salsa. Increase heat to medium-high and cook until the mixture begins to boil. Reduce heat to low and simmer until chicken is cooked, 3–5 minutes longer.

5 Meanwhile, heat taco shells as directed on package. Fill shells with chicken mixture, lettuce, tomatoes, sour cream, and cheese. Serve immediately.

Air-Fried Chicken Taquitos

AIR FRYING EVERYTHING

An air fryer can be your best friend in the kitchen, helping you to avoid high-fat or greasy meals. Air fryers use significantly less oil and don't produce the same harmful compounds as deep frying, so you can still eat your favorite foods but with fewer calories and less fat. Air fryers can be used for much more than frying. They can be used to hard-cook eggs, roast nuts, and even cook pizza!

Air frying makes these taquitos just as crunchy as the deep-fried kind. Feel free to add sour cream and a mild salsa for serving.

1½ cups shredded cooked chicken breast

2 teaspoons low-sodium taco seasoning

¾ cup shredded Monterey jack cheese

12 (6") corn tortillas

3 tablespoons olive oil

1   Toss chicken, taco seasoning, and cheese together in a large bowl.
2   Preheat an air fryer to 370°F.
3   Place a tortilla on a work surface and spread a generous 2 tablespoons filling across the middle of tortilla.
4   Roll tortilla around filling to form a cigar shape, securing with a toothpick if necessary to keep the tortilla rolled. Repeat this process with the remaining tortillas and filling. Brush the outsides of the taquitos with oil.
5   Place four taquitos in a single layer in the tray of the air fryer. Cook for 6 minutes, turning halfway through cooking time. Transfer to a plate, cover, and keep warm. Repeat the cooking process with the remaining taquitos. Serve hot.

Avocado Chicken Lettuce Wraps with Strawberry Relish

Mashed avocado provides a fresh take on traditional mayonnaise-laden chicken salad. Topped with a bright and sweet strawberry relish, this is a deliciously satisfying lunch that packs a hefty protein punch.

1 medium avocado, peeled, pitted, and chopped

3 tablespoons lemon juice

1 (5-ounce) can organic roasted chicken breast

1/4 teaspoon salt

1/4 teaspoon ground black pepper

3 tablespoons minced red onion

4 large strawberries, stemmed and diced

3 tablespoons chopped fresh cilantro

4 large Boston lettuce leaves

SERVES 2	
Calories	242
Fat	13g
Sodium	352mg
Carbohydrates	7g
Fiber	5g
Sugar	1g
Protein	24g

1 In a large bowl, use a fork to mash together avocado, lemon juice, and chicken. Season with salt and pepper.

2 Stir together onion, strawberries, and cilantro in a small bowl.

3 Place lettuce leaves on a large serving platter. Spoon chicken mixture into lettuce leaves and top with strawberry relish. Serve immediately.

Slow Cooker Chicken Chili Verde

SERVES 8	
Calories	340
Fat	8g
Sodium	813mg
Carbohydrates	27g
Fiber	8g
Sugar	8g
Protein	40g

No time? No problem! Let the slow cooker do the work for you in this protein-packed Southwestern dish. If beans cause digestion issues, try eating this meal earlier in the day.

½ tablespoon olive oil

2 pounds boneless, skinless chicken breasts, cut into 1" cubes

2 (28-ounce) cans whole peeled tomatoes, undrained

1 (16-ounce) can chili beans, drained and rinsed

1 (15-ounce) can kidney beans, drained and rinsed

1 (4-ounce) can diced green chili pepper, undrained

1 tablespoon Italian seasoning

1 tablespoon chili powder

2 teaspoons ground cumin

1 tablespoon granulated sugar

1 medium yellow onion, peeled and minced

3 cloves garlic, peeled and minced

½ cup water

¼ cup sour cream

1 Heat oil in a large skillet over medium-high heat. Add chicken and cook, stirring frequently, until browned on all sides, about 1–2 minutes per side. Transfer chicken to a greased 4–6-quart slow cooker.

2 Add the remaining ingredients (except sour cream) over chicken in the slow cooker.

3 Cover and cook on high for 3 hours or on low for 6 hours.

4 Uncover and stir to combine ingredients. Garnish with sour cream before serving.

Slow Cooker Chicken Cacciatore

This dish pairs well with spaghetti squash or zucchini noodles. If you have leftovers, put the zucchini noodles or spaghetti squash and the chicken mixture in different containers. When ready to eat, combine them and heat them in a saucepan over low heat.

SERVES 6	
Calories	380
Fat	18g
Sodium	721mg
Carbohydrates	14g
Fiber	3g
Sugar	8g
Protein	40g

2 pounds bone-in chicken thighs

1½ cups no-sugar-added marinara sauce

1 (6-ounce) can tomato paste

1 medium green bell pepper, seeded and diced

8 ounces sliced white mushrooms

1 yellow onion, peeled and diced

3 tablespoons minced garlic

1 teaspoon dried oregano

⅛ teaspoon crushed red pepper flakes

1 Place chicken in a 4–6-quart slow cooker. Top with remaining ingredients.

2 Cover and cook on low for 8 hours. Uncover and let cool for 5 minutes before serving.

Kung Pao Chicken

This recipe requires minimal cooking skills. Mix all of the ingredients together in a skillet for a super-easy flavorful and protein-rich dinner.

SERVES 6	
Calories	240
Fat	8g
Sodium	441mg
Carbohydrates	4g
Fiber	2g
Sugar	1g
Protein	38g

6 (4-ounce) boneless, skinless chicken breasts, cut in strips

4 cups broccoli florets

1 teaspoon sesame oil

1 clove garlic, peeled and minced

½ teaspoon all-purpose seasoning

2 tablespoons ground ginger

¼ teaspoon crushed red pepper flakes

1 cup low-sodium chicken broth

1 cup water

3 tablespoons hoisin sauce

3 tablespoons rice wine vinegar

3 tablespoons low-sodium soy sauce

¼ cup roasted, unsalted peanuts

1 teaspoon cornstarch

1 Mix all ingredients in a large bowl.

2 Spray a large skillet or wok with nonstick cooking spray and heat over medium-high heat. Add chicken mixture to skillet. Sauté for 10 to 15 minutes, stirring often. Serve immediately.

Slow Cooker Tangy Orange Chicken

SERVES 8

Calories	323
Fat	7g
Sodium	636mg
Carbohydrates	12g
Fiber	2g
Sugar	7g
Protein	53g

CAULI RICE IS HERE TO STAY

Cauliflower rice, a low-carb alternative to traditional rice, is made from finely chopped cauliflower. To make it at home, add chopped cauliflower florets to a food processor and pulse until they resemble grains of rice. Cauliflower rice can be sautéed in a hot skillet or simply heated in the microwave. The beauty of cauliflower rice is in its mild flavor that provides a neutral background for most flavors and dishes.

You can find prepared cauliflower "rice" in the produce section or in the frozen vegetable aisle in your grocery store. Or you can easily make your own.

3 pounds boneless, skinless chicken breasts

1 small yellow onion, peeled and diced

1/2 cup orange juice

3 tablespoons orange marmalade

1 tablespoon honey

1 tablespoon lemon juice

1 teaspoon Dijon mustard

1/2 teaspoon dried thyme

1/2 teaspoon garlic flakes

1 tablespoon arrowroot powder

4 cups cooked cauliflower rice

1 Grease a 4–6-quart slow cooker with nonstick cooking spray. Add chicken and onion to the slow cooker.
2 In a small bowl, mix together orange juice, marmalade, honey, lemon juice, mustard, thyme, and garlic flakes. Pour over chicken and cover. Cook on low for 6 hours or until chicken is cooked through.
3 About 10 minutes before serving, combine arrowroot with 2 tablespoons hot water in a small bowl. Add arrowroot mixture to the slow cooker and whisk to combine. Leave the slow cooker uncovered, turn the temperature to high, and continue to cook for 10 minutes to thicken the sauce. Serve over cauliflower rice.

Instant Pot® Chicken with Mustard and Apples

Apples are considered a low-glycemic food. They sweeten up a dish without spiking your blood sugar.

4 (6-ounce) skinless, bone-in chicken thighs

1/4 teaspoon ground black pepper

1/2 teaspoon salt, divided

1 tablespoon olive oil

1 large shallot, peeled and minced

2 cloves garlic, peeled and chopped

1 large Gala apple, peeled, cored, and thinly sliced

1/2 cup dark beer

1 tablespoon all-purpose flour

1/2 cup low-sodium chicken broth

2 tablespoons honey

1 tablespoon whole-grain mustard

1/2 teaspoon finely chopped fresh thyme

1/2 teaspoon finely chopped fresh sage

SERVES 4	
Calories	366
Fat	17g
Sodium	413mg
Carbohydrates	17g
Fiber	1g
Sugar	13g
Protein	36g

AN APPLE A DAY

Apples are an excellent food choice. They are high in fiber and have a low glycemic index, and eating the skin provides polyphenols, which help protect insulin-producing cells and promote insulin sensitivity.

1 Press the Sauté button on an Instant Pot®. Sprinkle chicken with pepper and 1/4 teaspoon salt.

2 When the Instant Pot® is hot, add chicken and sear on both sides, about 10 minutes total. Transfer chicken to a plate. Add oil to the pot. Add shallot and garlic and sauté for 2 minutes.

3 Return chicken to the pot and add apple and beer. Press the Cancel button. Close lid, press the Manual or Pressure Cook button, and adjust time to 10 minutes.

4 When the timer beeps, quick-release the pressure until the float valve drops. Press the Cancel button and open lid. Press the Sauté button.

5 In a small bowl, whisk flour and broth until smooth. Add broth mixture to the pot along with honey, mustard, thyme, sage, and remaining 1/4 teaspoon salt. Bring to a simmer and cook for 5 minutes.

6 Transfer to a serving platter and serve hot.

Quick Curry Chicken

Easy is the name of the game with this Indian-inspired recipe. Bamboo shoots and water chestnuts are low-glycemic ingredients that will soak up the bold flavors of the dish.

SERVES 2	
Calories	455
Fat	21g
Sodium	621mg
Carbohydrates	11g
Fiber	2g
Sugar	3g
Protein	55g

WHAT ARE BAMBOO SHOOTS?

Bamboo shoots are the edible portion of bamboo. They're often found canned or dried, and they can add a great crunch to your dish. They are high in fiber and vitamin E and low in calories. Enjoy them in stir-fries, soups, or salads, or even pickled.

2 tablespoons vegetable oil

1½ teaspoons minced fresh ginger

1 clove garlic, peeled and minced

1 tablespoon curry powder

2 (6-ounce) boneless, skinless chicken breasts, cut into 1" cubes

1 (8-ounce) can bamboo shoots, drained

1 (8-ounce) can water chestnuts, drained

2 teaspoons soy sauce

¼ cup low-sodium chicken broth

2 scallions, trimmed and sliced

1 Heat oil in a wok or large skillet over medium-high heat. Add ginger, garlic, and curry powder. Stir-fry until fragrant, 1–2 minutes. Add chicken and stir-fry for 5 minutes or until chicken is well mixed with the curry mixture. Remove from wok and set aside.

2 Add bamboo shoots, water chestnuts, and soy sauce to the wok. Cook for 1–2 minutes until bamboo shoots and water chestnuts are heated through and coated in curry mixture.

3 Return chicken to the wok and add broth. Bring to a boil, cover, and reduce heat to medium-low. Simmer for 4 minutes or until everything is cooked through. Garnish with scallions before serving.

Ground Turkey and Zucchini Rice Bowl

This rice bowl is a light, low-carb meal option for any time of the day! Ground turkey is one of the leanest cuts of meat you can cook with. If you're looking to increase your calories, be generous with the ranch dressing.

SERVES 6	
Calories	272
Fat	14g
Sodium	485mg
Carbohydrates	4g
Fiber	1g
Sugar	1g
Protein	32g

1 tablespoon olive oil

1 teaspoon minced garlic

1 medium yellow onion, peeled and diced

1½ pounds ground turkey

1 large zucchini, trimmed, quartered, and sliced

1 (10-ounce) package frozen cauliflower rice

1 teaspoon garlic powder

1 teaspoon onion powder

1 teaspoon salt

1 teaspoon ground black pepper

½ teaspoon paprika

1 teaspoon dried parsley

6 tablespoons Tessemae's Organic Habanero Ranch Dressing

1 Heat oil in a medium skillet over medium heat.

2 Add minced garlic and cook for 1 minute. Add diced onion and cook for an additional 4 minutes or until onion is softened. Crumble in turkey and cook, stirring, until no longer pink, about 7 minutes.

3 Stir in zucchini and cauliflower rice. Sprinkle garlic powder, onion powder, salt, pepper, paprika, and parsley on top and stir to combine. Cover and cook until cauliflower rice is softened, about 5 minutes.

4 Remove from heat and transfer to bowls. Drizzle each serving with 1 tablespoon dressing and serve.

Deconstructed Stuffed Pepper Bowls

SERVES 6	
Calories	273
Fat	15g
Sodium	675mg
Carbohydrates	10g
Fiber	3g
Sugar	5g
Protein	25g

This is a great recipe for meal prep. After step 3, divide the mixture among six containers. When you're ready to eat, microwave one serving for 2 minutes on high, then top with cheese.

2 tablespoons olive oil

1 small yellow onion, peeled and diced

2 cups chopped red bell pepper

1 teaspoon minced garlic

1 pound ground turkey

1 teaspoon salt

1/2 teaspoon ground black pepper

1 1/2 teaspoons chili powder

1 1/2 teaspoons ground cumin

1/2 teaspoon paprika

1 teaspoon dried parsley

1 tablespoon tomato paste

1 (14.5-ounce) can fire-roasted diced tomatoes

2 (10-ounce) packages frozen cauliflower rice

1 cup shredded Cheddar cheese

1 Heat oil in a large skillet over medium heat. Add onion and bell pepper and cook until softened, about 5 minutes. Add garlic and cook for 1 more minute.

2 Crumble turkey into skillet and cook, stirring, for 2 minutes. Sprinkle with salt, black pepper, chili powder, cumin, paprika, and parsley. Cook, stirring, until turkey is no longer pink, about 5 more minutes.

3 Stir in tomato paste and diced tomatoes. Add cauliflower rice and stir to combine. Cover and cook until softened, about 7 minutes.

4 Sprinkle cheese on top and stir until melted, about 3 minutes.

5 Serve immediately.

Deli Turkey Cobb Salad with Vinaigrette

If you've never made your own salad dressing, this is a good one to try. It's a basic vinaigrette, and it works well with any type of green salad. It's so easy to make, there's no need to buy store-bought dressings, which are often high in fat, sodium, and sugar.

1/4 cup apple cider vinegar

2 tablespoons lemon juice

1 teaspoon honey

1/2 teaspoon salt

1/2 teaspoon cracked black pepper

1 tablespoon Dijon mustard

2/3 cup extra-virgin olive oil

6 cups chopped romaine hearts

3/4 pound honey-roasted turkey breast, diced

3/4 pound deli ham, diced

1/2 cup cooked bacon crumbles

3/4 cup blue cheese crumbles

3/4 cup diced tomatoes

3/4 cup diced hard-boiled eggs

1 Combine vinegar, lemon juice, honey, salt, pepper, and mustard in a container or jar with a cover, place cover securely, and shake vigorously to combine. Add oil, cover again, and shake until emulsified.

2 Place romaine in a large salad bowl or on a large serving platter. Arrange turkey, ham, bacon, cheese, tomatoes, and eggs on top of the lettuce in neat rows. Drizzle with dressing before serving.

SERVES 8	
Calories	373
Fat	29g
Sodium	1,132mg
Carbohydrates	5g
Fiber	1g
Sugar	3g
Protein	23g

BATTLE OF THE SALAD GREENS

Both romaine lettuce and iceberg lettuce are low in calories and have a high water content. They have similar nutrition profiles, but romaine has more folate and vitamin K, while iceberg has more vitamin A. Iceberg leaves are more tender, so they are better for using as wraps, but romaine leaves are sturdier and better for heartier salads.

Greek Turkey Patties

Using ground turkey instead of beef makes these burgers leaner and easier on the stomach. Feta and olives pack in anti-inflammatory fats and provide a fun Mediterranean flavor profile. Serve the patties with a lettuce wrap or on a low-carb bun.

SERVES 6	
Calories	396
Fat	27g
Sodium	588mg
Carbohydrates	2g
Fiber	0g
Sugar	0g
Protein	36g

1½ pounds ground turkey

1½ cups crumbled feta cheese

1 clove garlic, peeled and minced

¼ cup low-sodium chicken broth

½ cup minced Kalamata olives

2 teaspoons Greek seasoning

½ teaspoon ground black pepper

2 tablespoons avocado oil

1 Combine turkey, cheese, garlic, broth, olives, Greek seasoning, and pepper in a medium bowl. Use your hands to mix until incorporated. Form into six patties.

2 Heat oil in a medium skillet over medium heat. Transfer patties to hot pan and cook for 5 minutes on each side, or until turkey is cooked through.

3 Serve immediately or transfer each burger to a separate airtight container and store in the refrigerator until ready to eat, up to one week.

IT'S ALL GREEK TO ME

The Mediterranean diet is renowned for its abundance of antioxidants and healthy fats, along with its benefits for heart health and weight management. However, it's not just about the food. The diet also encourages moderate consumption of red wine and emphasizes enjoying meals with friends. It highlights the slower pace of life practiced in Mediterranean countries.

Low-Carb Cabbage Wrap Street Tacos

This lower-carb version of a street food favorite is a great set-it-and-forget-it meal! Start it in the morning and it will be ready at dinnertime. If you're not a cabbage fan, use lettuce as a wrap instead.

1/2 pound grass-fed beef roast

2 tablespoons chopped garlic

1 small jalapeño pepper, seeded and diced (optional)

1 (14.5-ounce) can diced tomatoes

2 tablespoons olive oil

8 large green cabbage leaves

1/2 medium cucumber, diced

2 scallions, trimmed and minced

1 Place beef, garlic, jalapeño, tomatoes, and oil in a 4–6-quart slow cooker. Cover and cook on low for 8 hours. Transfer beef to a cutting board and shred with two forks.

2 Divide shredded beef among cabbage leaves and top with cucumber and scallions. Serve immediately.

SERVES 4	
Calories	251
Fat	11g
Sodium	144mg
Carbohydrates	7g
Fiber	1g
Sugar	3g
Protein	31g

PICK YOUR PEPPER

If you want the flavor of a pepper without the spice, there are plenty of alternatives. Anaheim peppers are milder than jalapeños but share a similar shape and texture. For a sweeter option, consider banana peppers, some of which have no heat at all!

Steak Salad with Blue Cheese and Walnuts

Every calorie counts! This savory salad is a protein powerhouse that packs in loads of calories, fiber, and nutrients. Top it with your favorite Italian dressing for a light and tasty meal.

SERVES 8	
Calories	176
Fat	11g
Sodium	379mg
Carbohydrates	5g
Fiber	2g
Sugar	3g
Protein	14g

STORING SALADS

Here are a few important tips for storing salads as leftovers: If possible, leave off any dressing until you are ready to serve. Use an airtight container, and place a paper towel in the container to absorb moisture. Try to eat the leftovers within 1–2 days for the best taste and texture.

1 teaspoon dried oregano

1 clove garlic, peeled and crushed

¼ teaspoon ground black pepper

1¼ pounds beef sirloin steak (1" thick)

¼ teaspoon salt

1 large head romaine lettuce

½ cup crumbled blue cheese

¼ cup chopped red onion

¼ cup toasted chopped walnuts

½ cup prepared Italian balsamic salad dressing

1 Preheat broiler.

2 In a small bowl, combine oregano, garlic, and pepper. Press mixture into both sides of steak, distributing mixture evenly.

3 Broil steak for 5–6 minutes per side. Transfer to a cutting board and let sit for 5 minutes. Season steak with salt and slice across the grain into ¼"-thick strips.

4 Slice lettuce across the rib into 1" slices and place in a large bowl. Add steak, cheese, onion, walnuts, and dressing. Toss to coat, and serve immediately.

Orange Beef and Broccolini Stir-Fry

Enjoy this healthier twist on a classic Chinese-American sweet and sour dish! This adaptation of the recipe uses petite, tender broccolini, which has a milder taste than broccoli.

2 large navel oranges

3 tablespoons soy sauce

1 tablespoon rice wine vinegar

1 tablespoon cornstarch

1 teaspoon agave syrup

1 tablespoon sesame oil, divided

6 cloves garlic, peeled and minced

2 tablespoons minced fresh ginger

1 pound beef sirloin, trimmed and cut into $1/8$" × 3" slices

2 pounds broccolini, cut into small florets

$1/3$ cup water

$1/2$ cup chopped scallions

1 Cut zest from oranges in wide strips, taking care not to include white pith. Julienne zest thinly and set aside. Squeeze juice from oranges into a small bowl. Add soy sauce, vinegar, cornstarch, and agave syrup and whisk to mix.

2 Heat $1/2$ tablespoon oil in large wok or skillet over medium-high heat. Add garlic and ginger; stir-fry for 2 minutes. Add beef; stir-fry for 3–4 minutes until browned. Remove beef from wok with a slotted spoon and set aside.

3 Add the remaining $1/2$ tablespoon oil to the wok and add broccolini. Stir-fry for 1 minute, then add water. Cover and reduce heat to medium-low. Simmer, stirring occasionally, until water evaporates and broccolini is tender, about 3 minutes.

4 Return beef to skillet along with orange juice mixture. Stir-fry until sauce has thickened, about 2–3 minutes. Top with julienned orange peel. Serve immediately.

SERVES 6	
Calories	213
Fat	11g
Sodium	91mg
Carbohydrates	10g
Fiber	5g
Sugar	4g
Protein	19g

BROCCOLI'S TALL COUSIN

Broccolini is a cruciferous vegetable, just like broccoli, and is a cross between regular broccoli and Chinese kale. Broccolini has a milder flavor compared to broccoli, with stems that are more tender and don't need to be peeled. This means that you don't need to cook broccolini as long as broccoli, but you can still substitute one for the other.

Steak and Veggie Stir-Fry

SERVES 4	
Calories	237
Fat	11g
Sodium	471mg
Carbohydrates	7g
Fiber	2g
Sugar	2g
Protein	27g

Top round steak is a lean, mild-tasting source of protein that pairs perfectly with fresh vegetables and a bright Asian-inspired stir-fry sauce.

3/4 pound top round steak, trimmed and cut in thin strips

2 tablespoons red wine vinegar

2 tablespoons olive oil, divided

1 tablespoon sliced fresh ginger

2 cups chopped broccolini

8 ounces white mushrooms, sliced

1 large carrot, peeled and sliced

1 cup low-sodium beef broth

2 tablespoons cornstarch

1 tablespoon soy sauce

1/8 teaspoon ground black pepper

1 Place steak in a shallow dish and sprinkle with vinegar and 1 tablespoon oil. Marinate for 10 minutes.

2 In a large skillet or wok, heat the remaining 1 tablespoon oil over medium-high heat. Remove steak from dish, reserving marinade. Add steak to skillet; stir-fry for 3–4 minutes until browned. Remove steak from pan and set aside in a medium bowl or plate.

3 Add ginger to skillet; stir-fry for 1 minute. Add broccolini, mushrooms, and carrot. Stir-fry for 5 minutes. Return steak to pan.

4 Add broth, cornstarch, soy sauce, and pepper to reserved marinade and stir well. Add mixture to skillet and bring to a boil. Cook, stirring, for 1–2 minutes until sauce is thickened and beef and vegetables are tender. Serve immediately.

Tangy Sirloin Salad

This main-dish salad is savory, sweet, and lightly spicy all at once. Sirloin is a leaner cut of steak that will help you knock out those protein goals for the day.

1/2 cup fresh basil leaves

1 tablespoon chopped serrano chili (optional)

2 cloves garlic, peeled

2 tablespoons light brown sugar

2 tablespoons fish sauce

1/4 teaspoon ground black pepper

1/4 cup lemon juice

1 (1-pound) sirloin steak

1 inner stalk lemongrass, finely sliced

2/3 cup thinly sliced red onion

1 cup thinly sliced cucumber

1/2 cup chopped tomato

1/2 cup mint leaves

2 small heads Bibb lettuce, split into leaves

SERVES 4	
Calories	326
Fat	16g
Sodium	415mg
Carbohydrates	13g
Fiber	2g
Sugar	10g
Protein	32g

1 Preheat a gas or charcoal grill.

2 Combine basil, chili, garlic, sugar, fish sauce, pepper, and lemon juice in a blender and process until almost smooth; set aside.

3 Grill steak to medium-rare (about 4 minutes per side), or to your liking. Transfer steak to a platter, cover with foil, and let rest for 5–10 minutes before carving.

4 Slice steak across the grain into thin slices. Transfer slices and any juices from the platter to a large bowl. Add lemongrass, onion, cucumber, tomato, and mint. Drizzle with reserved dressing and toss to coat.

5 Place lettuce leaves on individual plates and top with steak mixture. Serve immediately.

Pan-Fried Flank Steak with Swiss Chard

SERVES 8	
Calories	274
Fat	17g
Sodium	695mg
Carbohydrates	4g
Fiber	2g
Sugar	1g
Protein	26g

Swiss chard contains an antioxidant known as alpha-lipoic acid that is known to lower glucose levels and increase insulin sensitivity. The leaves have a slightly bitter taste, which is tempered here by cooking with garlic-infused oil and butter.

1 (2-pound) flank steak

1½ teaspoons salt, divided

1½ teaspoons ground black pepper, divided

1 tablespoon olive oil

2 cloves garlic, peeled and minced

½ teaspoon crushed red pepper flakes

2 pounds Swiss chard, stems trimmed

1 tablespoon unsalted butter

1 tablespoon vegetable oil

1 Pat steak dry with paper towels. Rub all sides with 1 teaspoon salt and 1 teaspoon black pepper. Set aside.

2 In a large nonstick skillet over medium heat, heat olive oil until shimmering. Add garlic and crushed red pepper and cook, stirring constantly for 30 seconds, being careful not to burn garlic. Using tongs, add Swiss chard and stir into oil and garlic. Cover and cook for 5 minutes. Stir in butter and the remaining ½ teaspoon each of salt and black pepper. Transfer to a large bowl and keep warm.

3 Wipe out skillet and place over medium-high heat until very hot, about 5 minutes. Add vegetable oil and heat until shimmering. Carefully add steak and sear for 3–5 minutes on each side.

4 Remove to a platter. Tent with foil and let rest for 10 minutes before slicing across the grain into thin strips.

5 Serve sliced beef with pan juices and Swiss chard.

Bulgogi Lettuce Wraps

This high-protein, low-carbohydrate Korean dish is nourishing, gut-healthy, and delicious! Kimchi is a beloved Korean side dish made of fermented vegetables that serves up probiotics and fiber along with a tangy kick.

1/2 cup soy sauce

2 tablespoons dark brown sugar

1 tablespoon toasted sesame oil

1 tablespoon mirin

2 cloves garlic, peeled and roughly chopped

2 teaspoons grated fresh ginger

1 pound flank steak, cut into 1 1/2" cubes

1 small head red leaf lettuce, split into leaves

2 cups kimchi

6 radishes, trimmed and thinly sliced

3 scallions, trimmed and thinly sliced

2 medium red or green serrano chilis, sliced (optional)

SERVES 4	
Calories	302
Fat	13g
Sodium	2,271mg
Carbohydrates	16g
Fiber	5g
Sugar	10g
Protein	30g

1 Place soy sauce, sugar, oil, mirin, garlic, and ginger in a blender or food processor. Process until smooth.

2 Place steak in a large resealable plastic bag and pour soy sauce mixture over it. Refrigerate for 1 hour.

3 Preheat a gas or charcoal grill to medium-high heat.

4 Remove steak from marinade and thread on metal skewers. Grill for 8 minutes, turning every 2 minutes.

5 Serve steak wrapped in lettuce leaves and topped with kimchi, radishes, scallions, and chili slices.

FOOD SAFETY FIRST

When preparing a meal with raw vegetables, it's essential to prevent cross-contamination with raw meat. One helpful method is to create food safety zones on your countertop during prep and cooking. Designate one area exclusively for raw meat, ensuring that nothing else is placed there and that raw meat does not come into contact with other foods.

Teriyaki Beef Stir-Fry

SERVES 4	
Calories	376
Fat	18g
Sodium	958mg
Carbohydrates	23g
Fiber	3g
Sugar	14g
Protein	30g

Marinating is a simple way to add flavor and ease digestion when cooking beef. Opting for low-sodium soy sauce minimizes the bloating that can be common for GLP-1 users.

1½ tablespoons low-sodium soy sauce

1 tablespoon mirin

1 teaspoon granulated sugar

1 pound flank steak, trimmed and cut into thin strips

1 pound chopped broccolini

3 tablespoons vegetable oil, divided

1 tablespoon minced garlic

2 teaspoons minced fresh ginger

¼ cup teriyaki sauce

1. In a medium bowl, combine soy sauce, mirin, and sugar. Add steak strips and stir to coat. Marinate for 20 minutes.
2. Blanch broccolini in boiling water for 2–3 minutes, until bright green. Plunge broccolini into cold water to stop the cooking process. Drain thoroughly.
3. Heat 1½ tablespoons oil in a wok or large skillet over medium-high heat until it is nearly smoking. Add garlic and stir-fry for 10 seconds.
4. Drain steak and discard marinade. Add steak to the pan, laying it flat. Let sear briefly, then stir-fry for 2 minutes or until no longer pink. Remove and drain in a colander or on paper towels.
5. Heat the remaining 1½ tablespoons oil in the wok or skillet over medium-high heat. Add ginger and broccolini. Stir-fry for 1 minute.
6. Stir in teriyaki sauce and bring to a boil. Return steak slices to the pan. Cook and stir for another minute. Serve hot.

Philly Cheesesteak–Stuffed Peppers

Two classic dishes are combined in one fun, nutrient-dense meal! Replacing rice with riced cauliflower slashes the carbohydrates in this comfort food recipe.

SERVES 6	
Calories	520
Fat	31g
Sodium	699mg
Carbohydrates	12g
Fiber	3g
Sugar	5g
Protein	48g

3 tablespoons olive oil

1 medium yellow onion, peeled and diced

1$\frac{1}{2}$ cups sliced white mushrooms

2 cups cauliflower rice

1$\frac{1}{2}$ pounds sliced roast beef, chopped

1$\frac{1}{2}$ cups shredded provolone cheese

1$\frac{1}{2}$ cups shredded mozzarella cheese

$\frac{1}{2}$ teaspoon sea salt

$\frac{1}{4}$ teaspoon ground black pepper

3 medium red bell peppers, seeded and tops cut off

3 medium green bell peppers, seeded and tops cut off

$\frac{1}{2}$ cup water

1 Press the Sauté button on an Instant Pot® and heat oil. When oil is hot, add onion and mushrooms and cook until softened, about 5 minutes.

2 Transfer onion and mushroom mixture to a large bowl and add cauliflower, roast beef, cheeses, salt, and black pepper. Stir to combine.

3 Stuff an equal amount of roast beef mixture into each bell pepper. Press the Cancel button and remove insert. Clean Instant Pot® insert and pour water into pot. Place a trivet in the Instant Pot®.

4 Arrange bell peppers on trivet. Close lid, press the Manual or Pressure Cook button, and adjust time to 15 minutes.

5 When the timer beeps, let pressure release naturally, about 20 minutes. Open lid and allow peppers to cool for 5 minutes before transferring to a platter.

6 Serve immediately.

Pot Roast with Root Vegetables

SERVES 8	
Calories	465
Fat	14g
Sodium	810mg
Carbohydrates	35g
Fiber	5g
Sugar	11g
Protein	49g

This wholesome classic dinner features low-glycemic root vegetables like carrots and sweet potatoes. Swapping the traditional white potatoes for sweet potatoes adds a healthy dose of fiber and vitamin A.

2 tablespoons vegetable oil

1 (4-pound) beef chuck roast

1 teaspoon salt

1/2 teaspoon ground black pepper

1 1/2 cups tomato juice

1 tablespoon Worcestershire sauce

4 medium sweet potatoes, peeled and diced

8 medium carrots, peeled and chopped

2 medium yellow onions, peeled and sliced

1 In a Dutch oven, heat oil over medium heat. Add beef and brown well on all sides, about 8 minutes. Season with salt and pepper.

2 Pour tomato juice and Worcestershire sauce over meat. Bring to a boil, then reduce the heat to low. Cover and simmer for 2 hours.

3 Add sweet potatoes, carrots, and onions to the Dutch oven. Cover and simmer for an additional 1 1/2 hours, or until meat is fork-tender and vegetables are done.

4 Transfer meat and vegetables to a platter and serve with braising juices on the side.

Steak and Mushroom Kebabs with Cauliflower Rice

These skewers are impressive enough for a dinner party, but easy enough for a weeknight family grill night.

3 tablespoons olive oil

1/4 cup balsamic vinegar

1 tablespoon Worcestershire sauce

1/2 teaspoon salt

2 cloves garlic, peeled and minced

1/8 teaspoon ground black pepper

1 pound sirloin steak, cut into 1 1/2" cubes

3/4 pound whole white mushrooms

1 large zucchini, trimmed and thickly sliced

2 cups cooked cauliflower rice

1 Combine oil, vinegar, Worcestershire sauce, salt, garlic, and pepper in a large bowl. Add steak, mushrooms, and zucchini and toss to coat. Cover and marinate in refrigerator for 2 hours.

2 Preheat a gas or charcoal grill.

3 Alternate steak cubes, mushrooms, and zucchini slices on wooden or metal skewers. Grill for 4 minutes per side for medium-rare steak. Serve hot with cauliflower rice.

SERVES 3	
Calories	572
Fat	37g
Sodium	1,012mg
Carbohydrates	13g
Fiber	2g
Sugar	3g
Protein	46g

COOK MUSHROOMS PERFECTLY EVERY TIME

Cooking mushrooms without making them soggy or too chewy can be challenging. The key is to keep them as dry as possible. You can rinse them quickly under water, but avoid submerging them, and be sure to dry them thoroughly right away. To prevent sogginess, add salt after cooking, as this will dehydrate them.

Instant Pot® Italian Beef and Peppers

SERVES 8	
Calories	326
Fat	11g
Sodium	164mg
Carbohydrates	10g
Fiber	1g
Sugar	3g
Protein	46g

GO LEAN

Choosing leaner cuts of beef can benefit your long-term health by lowering the amount of saturated fat. Some of the leanest cuts include chuck roast, top sirloin, flank steak, and round steak. On the flip side, the fattiest cuts of beef include ribeye and prime rib. You can further reduce fat by trimming visible fat and draining any excess fat after cooking.

While this Chicago classic is typically served on a sub roll, skipping the bread makes this a hearty, low-carb meal. The juicy, tender beef has an amazing, addictive flavor!

2 tablespoons vegetable oil

1 (3-pound) beef chuck roast, halved

1 large yellow onion, peeled, halved, and sliced

2 medium red bell peppers, seeded and sliced

2 medium green bell peppers, seeded and sliced

1 (16-ounce) jar sliced pepperoncini, including juice

3 cloves garlic, peeled and quartered

1 cup low-sodium beef broth

1 teaspoon ground black pepper

1 Press the Sauté button on an Instant Pot® and heat oil. Add one roast and sear for 5 minutes on each side. Remove from pot and repeat with remaining roast. Return first roast to pot.

2 Add onion, bell peppers, pepperoncini, garlic, and beef broth to pot with roasts. Press the Cancel button. Close lid, press the Manual or Pressure Cook button, and adjust time to 40 minutes.

3 When the timer beeps, quick-release the pressure until the float valve drops. Press the Cancel button and open lid. Transfer roasts to a cutting board and let rest for 10 minutes. Thinly slice, then place slices in a large bowl. Use a slotted spoon to transfer onions and bell peppers to the bowl, then add 3 tablespoons pot liquid to the bowl. Sprinkle with black pepper and toss lightly together. Serve warm.

CHAPTER 7

Seafood

Salmon Salad with Spring Vegetables and Lemon Dill Vinaigrette

Salmon is rich in omega-3 fatty acids, which are healthy, anti-inflammatory fats. It's also quick to cook and a great option when you can't look at another chicken breast. The lemon dill vinaigrette is so good, you'll want to put it on everything!

SERVES 4	
Calories	334
Fat	18g
Sodium	792mg
Carbohydrates	11g
Fiber	1g
Sugar	1g
Protein	32g

IT'S A BIG DILL

Dill, which is in the same family as parsley, has a fresh and citrusy flavor. It typically pairs well with fish, vegetables, and creamy dressings. Dill can lose its flavor easily with heat, so for hot dishes it's best to add it at the end. If replacing with dried dill, use 1 teaspoon of dried dill for every 1 tablespoon of fresh dill.

2 (8-ounce) skin-on salmon fillets

1¾ teaspoons salt, divided

½ teaspoon ground black pepper, divided

8 asparagus spears, trimmed and cut into 1" pieces

1½ teaspoons olive oil

½ pound new potatoes, cut in half

4 cups water

1 tablespoon grated lemon zest

2 tablespoons lemon juice

½ tablespoon minced fresh dill

¼ teaspoon Dijon mustard

⅛ teaspoon granulated sugar

2 tablespoons grapeseed oil

1 medium, head butter lettuce, torn

1 Preheat oven to 400°F.
2 On a foil-lined rimmed baking sheet, place salmon fillets skin side down. Sprinkle with ¼ teaspoon salt and ¼ teaspoon pepper. Roast until pink and flaky, about 20 minutes. Remove from oven and, using a fish spatula, remove the skin. Set salmon aside to cool, then cut into large chunks.
3 On another rimmed baking sheet, add asparagus and toss with olive oil, ¼ teaspoon salt, and ¼ teaspoon pepper. Roast until asparagus is tender, about 15 minutes.
4 Meanwhile, bring water and 1 teaspoon salt to a boil in a medium saucepan over medium-high heat. Add potatoes and cook until easily pierced with a fork. Drain potatoes and cool for 15 minutes.
5 In a small bowl, whisk together lemon zest, lemon juice, dill, mustard, sugar, grapeseed oil, and ¼ teaspoon salt until well combined.
6 In a large bowl, place lettuce, salmon, potatoes, and asparagus. Drizzle with vinaigrette and serve immediately.

Salmon Cobb Mason Jar Salad

You can cook some fresh salmon fillets instead of using canned salmon if you prefer, or use another protein source instead, like canned tuna, chopped chicken, or air-fried tofu. If you're trying to increase your calories, be generous with the avocado, blue cheese, and dressing.

1/2 cup Tessemae's Organic Creamy Ranch Dressing

2 (6-ounce) cans wild Alaskan pink salmon, drained

1/2 cup chopped hard-boiled egg

1/2 cup chopped turkey bacon

1/2 cup chopped avocado

1/2 cup crumbled blue cheese

1/2 cup chopped grape tomatoes

1/4 cup minced red onion

4 cups chopped iceberg lettuce

SERVES 4	
Calories	432
Fat	34g
Sodium	788mg
Carbohydrates	6g
Fiber	2g
Sugar	2g
Protein	26g

1 Put 2 tablespoons dressing in the bottom of each of four quart-sized wide-mouthed Mason jars.

2 Layer 3 ounces salmon, 2 tablespoons hard-boiled egg, 2 tablespoons bacon, 2 tablespoons avocado, 2 tablespoons cheese, 2 tablespoons tomatoes, 1 tablespoon onion, and 1 cup lettuce in each jar.

3 Cover and refrigerate until ready to eat, up to one week.

4 When ready to eat, shake vigorously to combine ingredients and coat with dressing.

Salmon and Avocado Salad

SERVES 2	
Calories	595
Fat	49
Sodium	713 mg
Carbohydrates	14g
Fiber	9g
Sugar	2g
Protein	25g

This creamy, delicious salad is chock-full of nutrients and can be whipped up in minutes. Both salmon and avocados contain healthy omega-3 anti-inflammatory fats that will nourish you for hours.

¼ **cup cream cheese, softened**

2 **tablespoons extra-virgin olive oil**

⅛ **teaspoon salt**

2 **teaspoons lemon juice**

8 **ounces smoked salmon, chopped**

2 **large avocados, peeled, pitted, and cubed**

1 Put cream cheese, oil, salt, and lemon juice in a food processor or blender and process until smooth.

2 In a medium bowl, mix salmon and avocado, then toss in cream cheese dressing. Refrigerate until chilled, 30 minutes to an hour. Serve chilled.

Ancho-Rubbed Salmon with Avocado Salsa

This mouthwatering dish is loaded with protein! Even better, the salmon fillet only takes 6 minutes to cook. High-protein meals like this are essential for maintaining a healthy muscle mass and metabolism.

1 large tomato, diced

1 large avocado, peeled, pitted, and diced

2 tablespoons minced fresh cilantro

1 scallion, trimmed and thinly sliced

2 tablespoons lime juice

3/4 teaspoon salt, divided

1 tablespoon light brown sugar

2 teaspoons ground ancho chili powder

1/2 teaspoon ground black pepper

4 (6-ounce) skin-on salmon fillets

SERVES 4	
Calories	388
Fat	19g
Sodium	536mg
Carbohydrates	9g
Fiber	3g
Sugar	5g
Protein	44g

1 Preheat a gas or charcoal grill for direct grilling.

2 Toss tomato, avocado, cilantro, scallion, lime juice, and ½ teaspoon salt together in a medium mixing bowl. Set aside.

3 Mix sugar, chili powder, pepper, and remaining ¼ teaspoon salt together in a small bowl. Rub on tops and sides of salmon fillets.

4 Place salmon, skin side up, directly on preheated grill. Cook for 4 minutes. Use a spatula to carefully turn salmon skin side down. Grill for an additional 2 minutes or until meat flakes easily when tested at edges but is not quite cooked through. Slide a metal spatula carefully between skin and flesh of the fish—the fillets should come free easily, while the skins will stick to the grill. Transfer salmon to a platter.

5 Spread salsa on a platter or individual plates, place salmon on top, and serve.

Grilled Salmon with Roasted Peppers

SERVES 4	
Calories	264
Fat	16g
Sodium	402mg
Carbohydrates	4g
Fiber	1g
Sugar	3g
Protein	26g

The fresh ginger gives the marinade a warm and spicy flavor, but it's also a natural remedy for nausea. Adding it to a recipe can help to settle an upset stomach.

4 (4-ounce) salmon steaks

2 tablespoons low-sodium soy sauce

1 tablespoon grated fresh ginger

1 teaspoon sesame oil

2 large red bell peppers

1 tablespoon balsamic vinegar

1/2 teaspoon dried rosemary

1/4 teaspoon ground black pepper

1 Place salmon in a shallow dish. Mix together soy sauce, ginger, and oil; pour over salmon and cover both sides with marinade. Set aside.

2 Preheat broiler.

3 Place whole bell peppers on a baking sheet and broil for 25 minutes, turning often, until skins are charred. Let cool, then cut in half and remove seeds and ribs. Cut into thick slices and sprinkle with vinegar, rosemary, and black pepper. Set aside.

4 Heat a gas or charcoal grill to medium. Remove salmon from the marinade and grill for approximately 8 minutes on one side. Turn and grill on the other side until salmon is cooked and tender, about 4–5 minutes longer. Remove from heat.

5 Serve salmon steaks with roasted bell peppers.

Salmon with Fresh Ginger Sauce and Cauliflower Rice

Who says cooking has to be complicated? This simple and refreshing dish can be whipped up in no time. It's also a great dish for meal prep. Refrigerate the salmon, sauce, and rice separately and enjoy the leftovers cold or warmed in the microwave.

1 (¼") piece fresh ginger, peeled and minced

½ cup mayonnaise

2 teaspoons chopped fresh cilantro

2 tablespoons lime juice

6 (4-ounce) salmon steaks or fillets

1 teaspoon salt

½ teaspoon ground black pepper

3 cups cooked cauliflower rice

1 Preheat oven to 400°F.
2 Combine ginger, mayonnaise, cilantro, and lime juice in a bowl.
3 Place salmon on a large rimmed baking sheet lined with foil and brush with ¼ cup ginger sauce. Season with salt and pepper. Reserve the remaining sauce for serving.
4 Bake for 25 minutes.
5 Serve salmon with remaining ginger sauce and cauliflower rice.

SERVES 6	
Calories	386
Fat	29g
Sodium	658mg
Carbohydrates	4g
Fiber	1g
Sugar	2g
Protein	27g

HOW DOES GINGER HELP NAUSEA?

Ginger helps ease nausea by speeding up stomach emptying and preventing food from lingering too long. It contains anti-inflammatory compounds that relax the stomach muscles and promote smoother digestion. Additionally, ginger can reduce fermentation in the gut, which can cause bloating and gas.

Instant Pot® Salmon with Lemon and Dill

SERVES 4	
Calories	255
Fat	15g
Sodium	354mg
Carbohydrates	0g
Fiber	0g
Sugar	0g
Protein	30g

This quick recipe is light in calories and seasoning, making it a great option for those with sensitive stomachs. For an easy side dish, add sliced vegetables to the cooking liquid so they poach while the fish steams. Good vegetables to include are asparagus, green beans, and thin strips of red bell pepper.

1 cup water

4 (4-ounce) skin-on salmon fillets

1/2 teaspoon salt

1/2 teaspoon ground black pepper

3 tablespoons chopped fresh dill

1 medium lemon, thinly sliced

2 tablespoons unsalted butter, softened

1 tablespoon chopped fresh parsley

1 Add water to an Instant Pot® insert and place the rack inside.

2 Place salmon on rack. Season with salt and pepper and top each fillet with dill and 2 slices lemon. Close lid and set steam release to Sealing, then press the Steam button and adjust cook time to 3 minutes.

3 When the timer beeps, quick-release the pressure until the float valve drops. Press the Cancel button and open lid. Place salmon on a serving platter and top with butter and parsley. Serve immediately.

Shrimp Tacos with Creamy Slaw

If you're in a time crunch, this tasty shrimp taco recipe only takes a few minutes to throw together. Keep a bag of frozen shrimp in the freezer; it's an excellent source of lean protein that can help you to reach your protein goals.

1/4 cup light mayonnaise

1/2 cup plain nonfat Greek yogurt

1/4 cup chopped yellow onion

2 teaspoons minced fresh cilantro

1/4 teaspoon kosher salt

2 cups shredded green cabbage

1/4 cup lime juice

1 clove garlic, peeled and minced

1 tablespoon olive oil

1 pound large shrimp, shelled and deveined

4 (8") high-fiber, low-carb flour tortillas

1 cup chopped tomato

1/4 teaspoon ground black pepper

SERVES 4	
Calories	331
Fat	12g
Sodium	980mg
Carbohydrates	28g
Fiber	13g
Sugar	4g
Protein	27g

1 In a medium bowl, whisk together mayonnaise, yogurt, onion, cilantro, and salt. Stir in cabbage and place in refrigerator to chill.

2 In a large bowl, combine lime juice, garlic, and oil. Add shrimp and stir to combine. Cover and refrigerate for at least 1 hour.

3 Heat a large skillet over medium-high heat and spray with non-stick cooking spray. With a slotted spoon, remove shrimp from marinade, add to pan, and sauté until cooked through, about 3–5 minutes. Discard marinade.

4 While shrimp is cooking, warm tortillas for about 20 seconds in the microwave.

5 To assemble tacos, divide shrimp into four portions. Place a portion in center of each heated tortilla. Top with cabbage mixture and tomato. Sprinkle with pepper and serve.

SHRIMP SKILLS

If you're new to cooking shrimp, there's no need to be intimidated. Start by removing the head and legs if they are still attached. Grasp the shrimp at the head end and pull off the shell. Then, use a knife to make a shallow cut along the back of the shrimp, about 1/4" deep, and remove the black vein. Keep your peeled shrimp in a bowl of ice while you finish peeling the rest.

Jumbo Sweet and Spicy Shrimp Skewers

SERVES 2	
Calories	412
Fat	23g
Sodium	498mg
Carbohydrates	21g
Fiber	1g
Sugar	18g
Protein	30g

Grilled skewers of shrimp make a fun and tasty summer dish that's ready in no time. If you're using wooden skewers, soak them in water for 20 minutes to prevent burning.

2 tablespoons honey

1 tablespoon mild hot sauce

1 tablespoon lemon juice

1 teaspoon fresh thyme leaves

12 jumbo shrimp, peeled and deveined, with tails on

1 medium shallot, peeled and quartered

2 white asparagus spears, trimmed and cut into 3" pieces

3 tablespoons peanut oil

¼ teaspoon salt

¼ teaspoon ground black pepper

1 Combine honey, hot sauce, lemon juice, and thyme in a large bowl. Add shrimp, stir to coat, and cover. Refrigerate for 30 minutes. Remove shrimp from marinade and pat dry. Reserve marinade for glaze.
2 Preheat a grill or broiler on high.
3 Thread shrimp, shallot quarters, and asparagus pieces onto wooden or metal skewers, alternating shrimp and vegetables. Brush with oil and season with salt and pepper.
4 Grill or broil for about 2 minutes per side.
5 Brush honey glaze over shrimp. Cook for 1 minute more on each side. Serve hot.

Cajun Shrimp and Mango Salad

This simple salad will transport you to a tropical paradise! While mangoes are higher in carbohydrates than other fruits, this recipe balances the carbohydrates perfectly with protein, fat, and fiber to provide healthy, stable energy throughout the day.

1 pound large shrimp, peeled and deveined

2 teaspoons Cajun seasoning

3 tablespoons butter

2 cloves garlic, peeled and finely minced

2 cups diced mango

1 cup chopped celery

1 tablespoon lemon juice

4 cups torn romaine lettuce leaves

1 Place shrimp in a large bowl. Sprinkle with Cajun seasoning and toss to coat.

2 Melt butter in a large skillet over medium heat. Add garlic and shrimp to skillet. Cook, stirring frequently, for 3–4 minutes until shrimp just turns pink. Pour contents of the skillet into a large bowl.

3 Add mango and celery to shrimp. Drizzle lemon juice over salad. Toss to mix and coat. Split lettuce between four plates. Top with shrimp mixture and serve immediately.

SERVES 4	
Calories	201
Fat	10g
Sodium	787mg
Carbohydrates	8g
Fiber	1g
Sugar	6g
Protein	20g

CHOPPIN' MANGOES

To properly and safely cut a mango, stand the mango on one end and cut straight down the middle until you hit the pit. Slide your knife along the edge of the pit down one side and repeat on the other side. Cut vertical and horizontal lines into each mango half without cutting the peel. Flip the mango half inside-out and peel the squares of fruit flesh off the peel.

Avocado and Shrimp Salad

Creamy avocado and refreshing citrus bring out the sweetness of shrimp in a salad you'll want to have again and again. Grapefruit has a low glycemic index, making it a great addition to your GLP-1 diet.

SERVES 4	
Calories	271
Fat	14g
Sodium	1152mg
Carbohydrates	12g
Fiber	4g
Sugar	6g
Protein	24g

1 large red grapefruit

2 tablespoons olive oil

24 jumbo raw shrimp, peeled and deveined

¼ cup chopped scallions, divided

2 cloves garlic, peeled and minced

2 tablespoons dry white wine

½ teaspoon salt

½ teaspoon ground black pepper

8 ounces butter lettuce, torn into bite-sized pieces

1 medium avocado, peeled, pitted, and sliced

1 Cut grapefruit in half. Squeeze the juice from one half. Remove the peel from the remaining half and slice fruit into bite-sized pieces. Set juice and fruit aside.

2 Heat oil in a large skillet over medium-high heat. Add shrimp and 2 tablespoons scallions. Cook shrimp 1 minute per side. Add garlic, wine, salt, and pepper. Cook, stirring frequently, for 1 minute. Stir in grapefruit juice and cook for 1 minute more.

3 Arrange lettuce, avocado, and remaining 2 tablespoons scallions on salad plates. Top with shrimp mixture.

4 Drizzle the sauce from the skillet over salads and garnish with the reserved grapefruit pieces. Serve immediately.

GRAPEFRUIT-STATIN INTERACTION

If you take a statin for high cholesterol, consuming grapefruit or grapefruit juice can increase your risk of side effects from the drug. However, this is only a concern with certain statins. Grapefruit also can interfere with antidepressants, antihistamines, and immunosuppressants, among other medications. Check with your doctor to see if you should avoid grapefruit in your diet.

Pineapple Shrimp Fried Rice

Pineapple fried rice combines two favorite flavors: sweet and salty. Using half cauliflower rice and half brown rice reduces the total carbohydrates while maintaining the texture of traditional fried rice.

1 teaspoon olive oil

1½ pounds medium shrimp, peeled and deveined

1½ cups cauliflower rice

4 scallions, trimmed and chopped

1 small jalapeño pepper, seeded and chopped

1 tablespoon minced garlic

2 cups cold cooked brown rice

1 cup diced pineapple

2 tablespoons low-sodium soy sauce or coconut aminos

1 teaspoon fish sauce

1 Heat oil in a large skillet over medium heat.

2 Add shrimp and cook for 3–5 minutes, turning once, until just opaque; remove from skillet and set aside.

3 Add cauliflower, scallions, jalapeño, and garlic to the skillet. Sauté for 2 minutes, then add brown rice and pineapple.

4 Stir in soy sauce and fish sauce. Return shrimp to the skillet and cook, stirring constantly, for 2 minutes.

5 Serve hot or at room temperature.

SERVES 6	
Calories	270
Fat	10g
Sodium	396mg
Carbohydrates	25g
Fiber	2g
Sugar	3g
Protein	20g

HOW TO CUT A PINEAPPLE

To cut a pineapple, begin by slicing off the top and bottom to create flat surfaces. Stand the pineapple upright and carefully slice off the skin, following its shape. Use a small, sharp knife to remove any remaining "eyes." Next, cut the pineapple into quarters lengthwise and slice out the core. Finally, chop the fruit to your desired size.

Shrimp in Coconut Milk

SERVES 4	
Calories	351
Fat	26g
Sodium	686mg
Carbohydrates	11g
Fiber	1g
Sugar	3g
Protein	18g

This recipe features a lean protein for healthy muscle mass, cinnamon for blood sugar balance, ginger for reducing nausea, and coconut milk for extra fat and calories. It checks all the boxes!

1 bay leaf

1 teaspoon cumin seeds

1 (1") piece cinnamon stick

2 whole cloves

4 black peppercorns

1 (1") piece fresh ginger, peeled and sliced

4 cloves garlic, peeled

3 tablespoons vegetable oil

1 large red onion, peeled and minced

1/2 teaspoon ground turmeric

1 pound large shrimp, peeled and deveined

1 (14-ounce) can light coconut milk

1/2 teaspoon salt

1 In a spice grinder, roughly grind bay leaf, cumin, cinnamon stick, cloves, peppercorns, ginger, and garlic. Add 1 tablespoon water if needed to form a thick paste.

2 In a large skillet, heat oil over medium heat. Add ground spice mixture and sauté for 1 minute. Add onion and sauté for 7–8 minutes until golden brown.

3 Increase heat to medium-high and add turmeric. Add shrimp and sauté for 2–3 minutes, just until they turn pink.

4 Stir in coconut milk and salt. Reduce heat to medium-low and simmer for 10 minutes or until sauce starts to thicken. Remove from heat and serve hot.

Mahi-Mahi Tacos with Avocado and Fresh Cabbage

This light summer recipe will transport you to the beach! Mahi-mahi is a lean whitefish that is high in protein and easy to prepare, even for those who are newer to cooking.

1 pound mahi-mahi fillets

1/2 teaspoon salt

1/2 teaspoon ground black pepper

1 teaspoon paprika

1 teaspoon olive oil

4 (6") low-carb flour or corn tortillas

1 medium avocado, peeled, pitted, and diced

2 cups shredded green cabbage

2 small limes, quartered

SERVES 4	
Calories	249
Fat	9g
Sodium	432mg
Carbohydrates	15g
Fiber	5g
Sugar	2g
Protein	27g

1 Season fish with salt, pepper, and paprika. Heat oil in a large frying pan over medium heat. Sauté fish for 3–4 minutes on each side until it flakes easily with a fork. Roughly chop fish and set aside.

2 Heat a small skillet over medium-low heat. Place tortillas in the pan and cook for about 1 minute on each side to warm.

3 Divide fish among the tortillas; top with avocado and cabbage. Serve with lime wedges.

Fish en Papillote

Not in the mood to cook? Try this easy baked fish recipe for a light, nutrient-dense dinner. Tarragon has been found to improve insulin sensitivity, which can help regulate blood sugar levels and reduce the risk of insulin resistance.

SERVES 6	
Calories	245
Fat	14g
Sodium	215mg
Carbohydrates	6g
Fiber	1g
Sugar	2g
Protein	24g

WHAT IS TARRAGON?

Tarragon is an herb with an anise flavor and a hint of sweetness. It makes a great complement to fish dishes, and the flavor is brought out nicely by lemon. Tarragon is great for adding at any stage of the cooking process, all with different flavor results. If you can't find tarragon, you can substitute chervil or fennel.

6 (5-ounce) whitefish fillets

½ teaspoon salt

½ teaspoon black peppercorns

1 teaspoon dried tarragon leaves

1 medium yellow onion, peeled and thinly sliced

1 large zucchini, trimmed and thinly sliced lengthwise

3 medium carrots, peeled and thinly sliced lengthwise

4 cloves garlic, peeled and minced

1 medium lemon, thinly sliced

1 tablespoon chopped fresh parsley

1 tablespoon olive oil

2 tablespoons dry white wine

1 Cut six (12" × 16") sheets of parchment paper, fold in half into 12" × 8" rectangles, and cut half a heart shape with center of heart along fold.

2 Unfold into heart shapes. Place a fish fillet near the fold on one side of each heart. Sprinkle with salt, peppercorns, and tarragon.

3 Place onion, zucchini, carrots, garlic, lemon, and parsley on top of each fillet. Drizzle each with oil and wine. Fold one half of each heart over the food and seal by crimping the edges together. Place bundles on rimmed baking sheets.

4 Bake for 20 minutes or until paper bundles expand and turn brown; fish should flake easily when tested with a fork. Serve the bundles, warning your guests to be cautious of steam when they cut them open.

Baked Red Snapper Veracruz

This Mexican-inspired recipe is low in carbohydrates and bursting with zesty flavor. Red snapper is a fantastic source of omega-3 fatty acids, lean protein, selenium, and potassium. It's also low in sodium, which keeps the bloating at bay.

1 tablespoon olive oil

1/4 cup finely diced yellow onion

4 ounces canned whole tomatoes

1/2 medium jalapeño pepper, seeded and minced (optional)

2 tablespoons diced pimento-stuffed olives

1 tablespoon fresh cilantro

1 (6-ounce) skinless red snapper fillet

1/8 teaspoon coarse salt

1/4 teaspoon crushed red pepper flakes

1 Preheat oven to 400°F.
2 Heat oil in a large nonstick skillet over medium-high heat. Add onion and cook until soft, about 5 minutes, stirring frequently. Add tomatoes, jalapeño, olives, and cilantro. Bring to a simmer and cook for about 3 minutes until slightly thickened.
3 Lightly oil a small baking dish with nonstick cooking spray. Place fillet in the center of the dish and season with salt and crushed red pepper. Fold the tail section under to make the fish consistent in thickness. Pour tomato mixture evenly over fish. Cover dish with foil and bake for 10–12 minutes until fish is opaque and flakes easily when tested with a fork. Serve hot.

SERVES 1	
Calories	369
Fat	17g
Sodium	460mg
Carbohydrates	8g
Fiber	3g
Sugar	5g
Protein	46g

MERCURY MEMO

Nearly all fish contain some mercury from their water and food sources. However, for most people, the risk from mercury content is minimal. Certain fish—such as king mackerel, swordfish, shark, albacore tuna, and red snapper—have higher mercury levels that can be harmful to fetal development. Therefore, pregnant women should limit their consumption of these varieties.

Tilapia with Tomatoes and Olives

SERVES 6	
Calories	137
Fat	4g
Sodium	288mg
Carbohydrates	3g
Fiber	1g
Sugar	1g
Protein	22g

If you're not too experienced in the kitchen, this Mediterranean-style recipe is a great way to dip your toes into cooking with minimal prep and cook time. It's low in carbohydrates but high in protein—just the combination we're looking for.

1½ cups diced tomatoes

½ cup chopped yellow onion

½ cup halved green olives

1 clove garlic, peeled and minced

1 tablespoon olive oil

½ cup white cooking wine

½ teaspoon all-purpose seasoning

¼ teaspoon ground black pepper

6 (4-ounce) tilapia fillets

1 Preheat oven to 350°F.

2 Mix tomatoes, onion, olives, garlic, oil, wine, seasoning, and pepper in a medium bowl and set aside.

3 Spray a 9" × 13" baking dish with nonstick cooking spray. Place fillets in the pan. Pour tomato mixture over the fillets and cover with foil.

4 Bake for 15 minutes or until fish flakes easily.

Cilantro Citrus Caribbean Mahi-Mahi

This easy-to-make dish is bursting with citrus and tropical flavors. And best of all, it's a wonderful weeknight dinner that can be ready in 20 minutes.

1 tablespoon olive oil

1 clove garlic, peeled and minced

1/2 teaspoon all-purpose seasoning

1/2 cup sliced yellow onion

1/2 cup chopped fresh cilantro

2 teaspoons chopped fresh parsley

1/4 cup orange juice

1/4 cup lemon juice

1/2 teaspoon ground cumin

6 (5-ounce) mahi-mahi fillets

1 medium lemon, cut in wedges

1 Combine oil, garlic, seasoning, onion, cilantro, parsley, orange juice, lemon juice, and cumin in a shallow dish. Add fillets and turn to coat.

2 Spray a large skillet with nonstick cooking spray and heat over medium heat. Add fish mixture and lemon wedges to skillet.

3 Cover and cook for 10–12 minutes until fish flakes easily.

SERVES 6	
Calories	151
Fat	4g
Sodium	126mg
Carbohydrates	3g
Fiber	0g
Sugar	1g
Protein	26g

SUPER CILANTRO

Researchers have discovered that cilantro stimulates an enzyme that removes sugar from the bloodstream, which will complement the work of GLP-1 in the body. Make sure to use fresh cilantro, instead of dried, to get the most nutrients.

Lemon Dill Tuna Salad Lettuce Cups

This fresh and light wrap can work as a protein-rich lunch, snack, or dinner. Choose canned light or chunk light tuna, made from skipjack tuna, for the lowest mercury levels.

SERVES 4	
Calories	134
Fat	4g
Sodium	412mg
Carbohydrates	3g
Fiber	1g
Sugar	2g
Protein	21g

SHOPPING FOR CANNED TUNA

Canned tuna is an excellent protein source that supports weight loss due to its low fat and calorie content. It's also incredibly convenient, as it comes fully cooked. To keep calories and fat lower, choose tuna packed in water. If you need additional calories, opt for oil-based tuna.

1 cup plain low-fat Greek yogurt

3 tablespoons lemon juice, divided

1 tablespoon chopped fresh dill

2 (5-ounce) cans chunk light tuna in oil, drained

1 tablespoon minced shallot

2 tablespoons capers

2 stalks celery, diced

¼ teaspoon salt

⅛ teaspoon ground black pepper

8 large iceberg lettuce leaves

1 In a small bowl, whisk together yogurt, 2 tablespoons lemon juice, and dill.

2 In a medium bowl, stir together tuna, shallot, capers, celery, remaining 1 tablespoon lemon juice, salt, and pepper.

3 Place 2 lettuce leaves on each of four plates. Divide tuna mixture among lettuce leaves, and drizzle with yogurt sauce. Serve immediately.

Tuna and Egg Salad

This simple 2-minute recipe tops protein with more lean protein! Serve the salad in a lettuce or egg white wrap for the lowest carbohydrate option.

2 large hard-cooked eggs, peeled

1 (5-ounce) can water-packed light tuna

1/4 cup plain low-fat Greek yogurt

1/4 cup diced white onion

1/4 cup pickle relish

1/4 teaspoon salt

1/4 teaspoon ground black pepper

SERVES 2	
Calories	167
Fat	6g
Sodium	722mg
Carbohydrates	12g
Fiber	1g
Sugar	9g
Protein	16g

1 Put eggs in a medium mixing bowl and mash with a fork.
2 Add tuna and yogurt and mash together until ingredients are combined. Stir in onion, relish, salt, and pepper. Serve.

Tuna and Apple Salad

This classic tuna salad with a twist is crunchy and refreshing with every bite! It's a great option for refueling after a workout. It will replenish your carbohydrates, protein, and calories all at the same time.

1 (5-ounce) can water-packed chunk light tuna

2 tablespoons mayonnaise

1 medium red apple, cored and diced

1/2 medium red onion, peeled and minced

2 stalks celery, chopped

1 large hard-cooked egg, peeled and diced

3 large Boston lettuce leaves

SERVES 3	
Calories	202
Fat	10g
Sodium	425mg
Carbohydrates	11g
Fiber	3g
Sugar	6g
Protein	17g

1 In a medium bowl, mix tuna, mayonnaise, apple, onion, and celery. Fold in egg.
2 Place a scoop of tuna salad on each lettuce leaf and serve.

Mini Crab Cakes with Smoky Aioli

SERVES 2	
Calories	387
Fat	29g
Sodium	530mg
Carbohydrates	0g
Fiber	0g
Sugar	0g
Protein	31g

Crab cakes are easier to prepare than you think! Crab is high in omega-3 fatty acids, which are known to lower inflammation. GLP-1 medications are thought to lower chronic inflammation as well. Eating foods containing omega-3s increases the benefit.

1 (8-ounce) can jumbo lump blue crabmeat

2 large egg whites

1 teaspoon dried chives

1/4 cup plus 1 tablespoon mayonnaise, divided

2 teaspoons lemon juice

4 cloves garlic, peeled and minced

1 teaspoon tomato paste

1/2 teaspoon smoked paprika

1/8 teaspoon cayenne pepper

1 tablespoon olive oil

1 Combine crab, egg whites, chives, and 1 tablespoon mayonnaise in a large bowl and mix until combined. Form mixture into four patties.

2 Place remaining 1/4 cup mayonnaise, lemon juice, garlic, tomato paste, paprika, and cayenne in a food processor and process until smooth.

3 Heat oil in a large skillet over medium heat and cook crab patties for 10 minutes or until cakes are browned and heated through, flipping once.

4 Top crab cakes with aioli and serve immediately.

CHAPTER 8

Vegetarian

Saucy Kung Pao Tofu

SERVES 6	
Calories	183
Fat	13g
Sodium	85mg
Carbohydrates	6g
Fiber	2g
Sugar	3g
Protein	11g

CORNSTARCH SLURRY

When you mix water with cornstarch before adding it to your dish, you're making what's called a cornstarch slurry. This method to thicken sauces is used because adding cornstarch directly can cause it to clump. Once the slurry is added, heat activates the cornstarch, allowing it to absorb the water in the dish and thicken the sauce.

Draining tofu effectively is the key to getting it as crispy as possible! If you plan on cooking with tofu regularly, buy a tofu press. They're so much easier to use than the typical method of wrapping a block of tofu in paper towels and weighting it down with a heavy pot. Serve this saucy stir-fry over cauliflower rice.

3 tablespoons soy sauce

2 tablespoons rice wine vinegar or cooking sherry

1 tablespoon sesame oil

2 (14-ounce) packages firm or extra-firm tofu, drained, pressed, and cubed

2 tablespoons vegetable oil

1 large red bell pepper, seeded and chopped

1 large green bell pepper, seeded and chopped

2/3 cup sliced white mushrooms

3 cloves garlic, peeled and minced

3 small red or green chili peppers, seeded and diced

1 teaspoon crushed red pepper flakes

1 teaspoon ground ginger

1/2 cup vegetable broth

1/2 teaspoon granulated sugar

1 1/2 teaspoons cornstarch

1 tablespoon water

2 scallions, trimmed and chopped

1/2 cup roasted peanuts

1 In a shallow baking dish, whisk together soy sauce, vinegar, and sesame oil. Add tofu and toss to coat. Marinate in the refrigerator for at least 2 hours. Drain tofu, reserving marinade.

2 In a large skillet, heat vegetable oil over medium-high heat. Add bell peppers, mushrooms, garlic, chili peppers, and crushed red pepper. Sauté for 3 minutes. Add tofu and sauté for 1–2 minutes, until vegetables are tender.

3 Add reserved marinade, ginger, broth, and sugar. In a small bowl, combine cornstarch with water. Add cornstarch slurry to mixture in skillet. Reduce heat to low and simmer for 2 minutes, stirring constantly, until sauce thickens. Add scallions and peanuts and heat for 1 minute. Serve immediately.

Basil, Eggplant, and Tofu Stir-Fry

Tofu not only is a great source of protein but adapts easily to a variety of flavors, like this savory stir-fry sauce. If you have any left over, wrap it in a lettuce leaf or low-carb tortilla for a quick lunch the next day.

2 tablespoons olive oil

3 cloves garlic, peeled and minced

1 (14-ounce) package firm or extra-firm tofu, drained, pressed, and cubed

1 large eggplant, trimmed and chopped into 2" pieces

1 medium red bell pepper, seeded and chopped

1/3 cup sliced white mushrooms

3 tablespoons water

2 tablespoons low-sodium soy sauce

1 teaspoon lemon juice

1/3 cup fresh basil leaves

1 In a large skillet, heat oil over medium-high heat. Add garlic and tofu. Sauté for 4–6 minutes until tofu is lightly golden.

2 Add eggplant, pepper, mushrooms, water, and soy sauce. Cook, stirring frequently, for 5–6 minutes until eggplant is almost soft.

3 Add lemon juice and basil and sauté for 1–2 minutes until basil is wilted. Serve hot.

SERVES 3	
Calories	219
Fat	13g
Sodium	16mg
Carbohydrates	14g
Fiber	6g
Sugar	9g
Protein	12g

HERBS AT HOME

Have you ever tried growing your own herbs at home? Even if you don't have a green thumb, anyone can successfully grow their own herbs. A few common choices for beginners include basil, cilantro, parsley, mint, thyme, and rosemary. Plant seeds about 1/4" deep in soil and keep the soil moist but not soggy. In just 6–8 weeks, you could be cooking with your own fresh herbs!

Coconut Lime Tempeh Stir-Fry

SERVES 2	
Calories	341
Fat	15g
Sodium	41mg
Carbohydrates	28g
Fiber	12g
Sugar	10g
Protein	24g

Since it's hard to eat a large amount of food while you're taking GLP-1, the more variety you can consume, the better! This quick stir-fry recipe is a great opportunity to pack in a variety of vegetables and nutrients without filling you up too much. Serve with cauliflower rice to add one more vegetable to the mix.

1 tablespoon sesame oil

½ cup thinly sliced white onion

2 cloves garlic, peeled and minced

1 cup sliced button mushrooms

½ cup chopped red bell pepper

8 ounces organic tempeh, crumbled

2 cups fresh spinach leaves

2 tablespoons lime juice

2 tablespoons low-sodium soy sauce

2 tablespoons unsweetened shredded coconut

¼ teaspoon crushed red pepper flakes (optional)

1 Heat sesame oil in a large frying pan or wok over medium heat. Add onion, garlic, mushrooms, bell pepper, and tempeh; sauté for 5–7 minutes until onions are translucent and mushrooms soften.

2 Stir in spinach and lime juice and cook for 1–2 minutes until spinach wilts. Mix in soy sauce, coconut, and crushed red pepper; cook for about 1 minute until heated through. Serve warm.

Vegetarian Mapo Tofu

Mapo tofu is a popular Chinese dish that usually contains ground beef and tongue-tingling Sichuan peppercorns. This milder version is a protein powerhouse with both tofu and soy crumbles as lean protein sources. It's typically served over rice, but a low-carb option like cauliflower rice would work equally well.

SERVES 4	
Calories	213
Fat	15g
Sodium	93mg
Carbohydrates	7g
Fiber	2g
Sugar	4g
Protein	13g

3 tablespoons vegetable oil

4 cloves garlic, peeled and minced

1 (1") piece fresh ginger, peeled and thinly sliced

3 tablespoons black bean–garlic sauce

2 tablespoons low-sodium soy sauce

1 tablespoon garlic-chili paste

1 cup vegetable broth

1 tablespoon cornstarch

1 tablespoon granulated sugar

1 pound firm tofu, drained, pressed, and cubed

6 ounces soy "meat" crumbles

2 bunches scallions, trimmed and cut on the diagonal

1 Heat oil in a large wok or skillet over medium heat. Add garlic and ginger and stir-fry for 30 seconds. Stir in black bean–garlic sauce, soy sauce, and garlic-chili paste.

2 In a small bowl, whisk together broth, cornstarch, and sugar and add to the wok. Stir in tofu and soy "meat" and stir-fry until sauce thickens and tofu is heated through. Add scallions, stir-fry for 2 minutes more, and serve.

Kimchi Tofu Soup

Kimchi is a fermented food that contains natural probiotics to fuel the gut microbiome. This flavorful recipe is nourishing, light on the stomach, and rich in protein.

SERVES 4	
Calories	190
Fat	10g
Sodium	1,203mg
Carbohydrates	9g
Fiber	2g
Sugar	4g
Protein	16g

1 tablespoon peanut oil

2 tablespoons minced shallot

2 cloves garlic, peeled and minced

1 (3") piece fresh ginger, peeled and minced

1 tablespoon garlic-chili paste

¼ cup soy sauce

1 tablespoon rice wine vinegar

6 cups low-sodium vegetable broth

2 (14-ounce) packages firm tofu, drained, pressed, and cut into ½" cubes

1 cup kimchi

2 scallions, trimmed and sliced

1 Heat oil in a medium saucepan over medium-high heat. Add shallot, garlic, and ginger, and sauté until fragrant, about 4 minutes. Stir in garlic-chili paste, soy sauce, and vinegar. Add broth and bring to a boil.

2 Reduce heat to medium-low. Add tofu and simmer for 20 minutes. Stir in kimchi and cook, stirring occasionally, until heated through, about 5 minutes.

3 Top with scallions and serve.

THE GOOD BACTERIA FOR YOUR GUT

Have you heard that fermented foods are "good for you" but aren't sure why? The fermentation process naturally creates probiotics by using bacteria to break down sugars and starches, which creates an environment that promotes the growth of healthy bacteria. Popular fermented foods include kimchi, sauerkraut, kefir, and miso.

Lemon Tempeh with Zucchini Pasta in Sweet Honey Yogurt

Zucchini noodles are a fantastic lower-carb alternative to regular pasta. You can make your own or buy them premade at the grocery store. Add some lemon zest to the yogurt mixture for an extra burst of lemony flavor.

1 cup nonfat plain yogurt

1 tablespoon honey

2 large zucchini, trimmed

1 tablespoon olive oil

8 ounces tempeh, sliced or cubed

1 teaspoon salt

2 tablespoons lemon juice

1. In a large bowl, whisk yogurt and honey to combine.
2. Using a spiralizer, create noodles from zucchini and add noodles to the yogurt mixture.
3. Heat oil in a large skillet over medium heat. Add tempeh and cook for 3–5 minutes on each side until slightly browned.
4. Season tempeh with salt, then add lemon juice to skillet and cook for 2–3 minutes until slightly golden. Remove from heat.
5. Place equal amounts of zucchini noodles in each of two serving bowls and top with equal amounts of tempeh. Serve warm or chilled.

SERVES 2	
Calories	382
Fat	11g
Sodium	1,261mg
Carbohydrates	38g
Fiber	10g
Sugar	9g
Protein	32g

TIPS FOR COOKING TEMPEH

Before cooking with tempeh, you can microwave it with water for about 2 minutes to reduce its bitterness. Tempeh absorbs flavors well, so cut it into small cubes or thin slices to maximize the surface area. Finally, don't hesitate to experiment with seasonings; you can treat it just like meat when it comes to flavoring.

Air Fryer Curried Tofu and Turmeric Cauli Rice

SERVES 4	
Calories	222
Fat	13g
Sodium	300mg
Carbohydrates	17g
Fiber	6g
Sugar	1g
Protein	9g

This low-carb tofu dish is full of inflammation-fighting ingredients like avocado oil, coconut oil, and turmeric. Feel free to substitute premade cauliflower rice from the grocery store instead of making it from scratch.

8 ounces extra-firm tofu, drained, pressed, and cubed

½ cup canned unsweetened coconut milk

2 teaspoons red curry paste

2 cloves garlic, peeled and minced

1 tablespoon avocado oil

1 tablespoon coconut oil

1 small head cauliflower, pulsed into rice

1 tablespoon ground turmeric

½ teaspoon salt

½ teaspoon freshly ground white pepper

½ medium lime, cut into 4 wedges

¼ cup chopped fresh cilantro

1 In a medium bowl, combine tofu, coconut milk, curry paste, garlic, and avocado oil. Cover and refrigerate for 30 minutes.

2 Preheat an air fryer to 350°F.

3 Place tofu and marinade in an ungreased air fryer cake barrel. Place in air fryer basket and cook for 5 minutes. Stir, then cook for an additional 5 minutes.

4 While tofu is cooking, heat coconut oil in a medium skillet over medium-high heat. Add cauliflower, turmeric, salt, and pepper. Stir-fry for 6 minutes or until cauliflower is tender.

5 Add cauliflower rice to four medium bowls. Top with tofu mixture and sauce. Garnish with lime wedges and cilantro. Serve warm.

Air-Fried Tofu

The best way to make sure you are hitting your protein goals is to make sure you always have protein sources readily available. Prepare batches of this air fryer tofu ahead of time to throw into salads, pastas, stir-fries, and more!

1 (14-ounce) package extra-firm tofu, drained, pressed, and cubed

2 teaspoons olive oil

¼ teaspoon salt

SERVES 4	
Calories	118
Fat	7g
Sodium	149mg
Carbohydrates	3g
Fiber	1g
Sugar	0g
Protein	11g

1 Preheat air fryer to 375°F and set timer for 18 minutes.

2 Remove fryer basket and spray with nonstick cooking spray. Add tofu and oil. Toss to coat, then place basket back in air fryer.

3 Every 5 minutes, remove basket and stir tofu by shaking basket carefully. Cook until timer goes off and tofu is crispy. Remove from basket and sprinkle with salt.

4 Serve hot or at room temperature.

AIR FRYER TIPS

When using an air fryer, be sure to preheat it for even cooking. To achieve the best crispiness, avoid overcrowding the basket. Remember to shake or flip the food a couple of times during the cooking process. Make sure to clean the basket as soon as possible after cooking.

Lentil Salad with Roasted Vegetables

If you're looking for a meatless protein source, don't overlook lentils! They're rich in fiber and protein, and they add a lot of volume to this crunchy salad.

SERVES 4	
Calories	258
Fat	13g
Sodium	1,342mg
Carbohydrates	27g
Fiber	8g
Sugar	5g
Protein	8g

1 (1-pound) celery root, peeled and cubed

2 medium carrots, peeled and cut into 1" pieces

1 medium red onion, peeled and roughly chopped

¼ cup olive oil, divided

1 teaspoon ground black pepper

2 teaspoons salt, divided

2 cups vegetable broth

1 cup brown lentils, rinsed

2 tablespoons lemon juice

2 teaspoons ground cumin

½ teaspoon crushed red pepper flakes

2 tablespoons roughly chopped fresh parsley

1 Preheat oven to 400°F. Line a large baking sheet with parchment paper.

2 Toss celery root, carrots, and onion with 2 tablespoons oil in a medium bowl. Season with black pepper and 1 teaspoon salt. Spread vegetables out in a single layer on the prepared baking sheet and roast for 20 minutes, turning once halfway through.

3 Meanwhile, in a medium saucepan, bring broth and lentils to a boil over medium heat. Reduce heat to medium-low and simmer for 18–20 minutes or until cooked through. Drain in a colander.

4 Place lentils in a large bowl and stir in roasted vegetables. In a small bowl, whisk together lemon juice, cumin, crushed red pepper, and parsley with the remaining 2 tablespoons oil and 1 teaspoon salt. Pour over lentils and vegetables, and toss to combine.

Greek Pasta Salad

This Mediterranean-inspired pasta salad is an easy option for lunch or dinner. You'll get a double serving of protein and fiber from the pasta and the chickpeas.

SERVES 8	
Calories	426
Fat	22g
Sodium	955mg
Carbohydrates	26g
Fiber	15g
Sugar	4g
Protein	31g

½ cup extra-virgin olive oil

¼ cup balsamic vinegar

½ teaspoon salt

¼ teaspoon ground black pepper

1 (14.5-ounce) package high-protein rotini pasta, cooked according to package instructions

1 pint cherry tomatoes, halved

1 medium cucumber, peeled and diced

1 medium yellow bell pepper, seeded and diced

¼ small red onion, peeled and thinly sliced

1 cup canned chickpeas, drained and rinsed

1 cup crumbled feta cheese

½ cup sliced black olives

½ cup roughly chopped fresh mint leaves

1 In a small bowl, whisk together oil, vinegar, salt, and black pepper. Set aside.

2 In a large serving bowl, gently toss together pasta, tomatoes, cucumber, bell pepper, onion, chickpeas, feta, and olives.

3 Pour dressing over pasta mixture and toss well to coat. Garnish with mint. Serve immediately or refrigerate for up to three days.

Vegetarian Lasagna

SERVES 10	
Calories	329
Fat	8g
Sodium	552mg
Carbohydrates	50g
Fiber	8g
Sugar	9g
Protein	14g

This isn't your average lasagna! Lentils are a low-glycemic food that provides the texture of a meat, while kale is high in fiber, antioxidants, potassium, and other key nutrients.

1 pound whole-grain lasagna noodles

1 tablespoon olive oil

1 large eggplant, trimmed and cut in $1/4$"-thick slices

2 cloves garlic, peeled and minced

2 medium shallots, peeled and finely sliced

4 cups marinara sauce

1 cup cooked red lentils

1 cup steamed kale

1 cup shredded fontina cheese

$1/2$ teaspoon ground black pepper

1 Preheat oven to 350°F. Fill a large bowl with water and ice cubes.

2 Bring a large pot of water to a slow boil. Partially cook the pasta in boiling water for 4 minutes, then shock in ice water.

3 Heat oil in a medium skillet over medium heat. Sauté eggplant, garlic, and shallots for 4–5 minutes until soft.

4 Ladle enough sauce into a large ungreased baking dish to coat the bottom. Layer pasta sheets over the sauce, then top with layers of lentils, kale, eggplant mixture, cheese, and pepper. Ladle sauce over the top. Repeat layering until the pan is almost full, finishing with a top layer of pasta, sauce, and cheese.

5 Cover with foil and bake for 45 minutes or until dish is heated through and cheese is melted. Uncover and bake for another 15 minutes. Remove from oven and let stand for 10 minutes before serving.

White Bean Cassoulet

Cannellini beans, also known as white kidney beans, are loaded with fiber, which can help control blood sugar and cholesterol levels, among many other health benefits.

1 pound dried cannellini beans

1 teaspoon canola oil

2 large leeks, thinly sliced (white and pale green parts only)

1 cup crushed tomatoes

2 cups vegetable broth

1/2 teaspoon ground fennel

1 teaspoon fresh rosemary

1/8 teaspoon ground cloves

1/4 teaspoon kosher salt

1/4 teaspoon freshly ground black pepper

1 The night before making the soup, place beans in a 4- to 5-quart slow cooker. Fill with water to 1" below the top of the insert. Soak overnight.

2 Drain beans and return to the slow cooker.

3 Heat oil in a large nonstick skillet over medium-high heat. Add leeks and sauté for 1 minute until leeks begin to wilt. Add leeks to the slow cooker. Stir in tomatoes, broth, fennel, rosemary, cloves, salt, and pepper.

4 Cook on low for 8 hours.

SERVES 8	
Calories	82
Fat	1g
Sodium	254mg
Carbohydrates	14g
Fiber	3g
Sugar	1g
Protein	4g

WHY SOAK BEANS?

Soaking dried beans is an important step to make sure you get tender and evenly cooked beans. Some only need to be soaked for a few hours, but others, like white beans, need to be soaked overnight. If you have hard water, you may need to add additional time for cooking or soaking, because calcium can prevent beans from softening.

Soy Citrus Ginger Edamame

SERVES 4	
Calories	148
Fat	7g
Sodium	1,465mg
Carbohydrates	8g
Fiber	3g
Sugar	2g
Protein	13g

If you're looking for a snack to satisfy your salt cravings, try this flavorful edamame recipe. You'll be pleasantly surprised by the tangy orange sauce!

1 tablespoon vegetable oil

2 tablespoons minced fresh ginger

½ cup soy sauce

¼ cup rice wine vinegar

2 tablespoons orange juice

1 tablespoon grated orange zest

2 cups fresh or frozen edamame in the pod

1 Heat oil in a large skillet or wok over medium-high heat. Stir in ginger, soy sauce, vinegar, orange juice, and orange zest. Bring to a boil and reduce heat to medium-low. Stir constantly until the sauce has thickened, about 6 minutes.

2 Toss in edamame and cook until heated through and well coated in sauce, about 1–2 minutes for frozen edamame or 5–6 minutes for fresh.

Egg-Cellent Salad

SERVES 4	
Calories	218
Fat	14g
Sodium	170mg
Carbohydrates	4g
Fiber	0g
Sugar	3g
Protein	19g

This classic egg salad makes an easy low-carbohydrate snack or lunch throughout the week. If you consume eggs on a regular basis, search for pasture or free-range eggs to get the most bang for your buck with nutrients.

12 large hard-cooked eggs, peeled

1 cup chopped celery

½ cup chopped scallions

2 tablespoons white wine vinegar

¼ cup plain nonfat Greek yogurt

1 teaspoon garlic powder

2 teaspoons ground black pepper

1 Place eggs into a large dish and mash with a fork.

2 Gently fold in celery, scallions, vinegar, yogurt, garlic powder, and pepper.

3 Cover and refrigerate for at least 1 hour before serving.

Asian Cabbage and Edamame Salad

This Asian-inspired salad features a refreshing lime dressing that will keep you coming back for more. Edamame provides protein, while the cabbage and radishes add a crunchy burst of fiber and antioxidants.

1 (8-ounce) package frozen shelled edamame

8 cups shredded red cabbage

4 large radishes, trimmed and sliced

1/4 cup diced red onion

2 tablespoons roughly chopped fresh basil

2 tablespoons roughly chopped fresh cilantro

3 tablespoons olive oil

2 tablespoons tamari

2 tablespoons lime juice

1/2 teaspoon salt

1/2 teaspoon ground black pepper

1 teaspoon ground coriander

1 Place edamame in a small bowl with 1 tablespoon water. Microwave for 5 minutes on high, and drain in a strainer. Run under cold water and drain again.

2 Place edamame, cabbage, radishes, onion, basil, and cilantro in a large bowl and toss to combine.

3 In a small bowl, whisk together oil, tamari, lime juice, salt, pepper, and coriander. Drizzle over the salad and toss well to coat. Serve immediately.

SERVES 4	
Calories	241
Fat	14g
Sodium	666mg
Carbohydrates	18g
Fiber	8g
Sugar	8g
Protein	11g

WHAT IS TAMARI?

Tamari is a Japanese sauce that is made by cooking and fermenting soybeans. If this sounds similar to soy sauce, that's because it is! The difference is that wheat is added into the fermentation process of soy sauce. Tamari tastes slightly richer than soy sauce and has a thicker consistency, but it still makes a perfect gluten-free swap for soy sauce.

Cucumber and Edamame Salad

This sweet and savory salad will surprise your taste buds. If you're able to tolerate it, increase the amount of edamame in the salad to get you closer to your GLP-1 protein goals.

SERVES 2	
Calories	282
Fat	18g
Sodium	436mg
Carbohydrates	17g
Fiber	8g
Sugar	5g
Protein	13g

2 cups chopped cucumber

1 cup shelled edamame, cooked

1/2 medium avocado, peeled, pitted, and diced

1 scallion, trimmed and minced

2 teaspoons sesame seeds

1 teaspoon red miso paste

1/4 cup lemon juice

1 tablespoon sesame oil

1/2 teaspoon raw honey

1 Combine cucumber, edamame, avocado, scallion, and sesame seeds in a large bowl.

2 Whisk together miso paste, lemon juice, oil, and honey in a small bowl until smooth. Pour dressing into the large bowl and toss until everything is evenly coated. Serve immediately.

WHY SESAME OIL?

Sesame oil has a prominent, distinctive flavor. It's made from sesame seeds, which give it a nutty and earthy flavor. Sesame oil can be used for cooking, but its flavor will change under heat, so it's best used drizzled on at the end of cooking or on a salad.

Tofu Lettuce Wraps

This Korean-inspired recipe keeps the carbohydrates low but the flavor high. The tofu will soak up the variety of spices and flavors of the slightly spicy sauce. If gochujang paste is too spicy for you, you can replace it with miso paste.

2 tablespoons low-sodium soy sauce

1 tablespoon gochujang paste

1 tablespoon honey

1 teaspoon sesame oil

2 scallions, trimmed and sliced

1 (12.3-ounce) package firm tofu, drained, pressed, and cubed

2 tablespoons vegetable oil

1 small shallot, peeled and thinly sliced

1/2 tablespoon minced garlic

1 small red bell pepper, seeded and diced

1 cup shelled edamame

1/4 teaspoon ground black pepper

1/2 teaspoon toasted sesame seeds

8 large Bibb lettuce leaves

SERVES 4	
Calories	184
Fat	12g
Sodium	225mg
Carbohydrates	7g
Fiber	4g
Sugar	3g
Protein	12g

IMPORTANT TOFU TIP

The most important step in cooking tofu is to press it. Wrap the tofu in a kitchen towel, then put something heavy, like a cast iron pan or pot, on top, and let it sit for at least 30 minutes. This will get out any liquid so that the tofu can soak up your marinade and crisp up nicely.

1 In a medium bowl, whisk together soy sauce, gochujang paste, honey, sesame oil, and scallions. Stir in tofu and gently toss until coated. Refrigerate for 1 hour.

2 Heat oil in a wok over medium heat. Add shallot and garlic and cook for 30 seconds. Toss in bell pepper and edamame and stir-fry for 2 minutes.

3 Add tofu with marinade. Stir-fry for an additional 2 minutes and sprinkle with black pepper and sesame seeds.

4 Place 2 lettuce leaves on each of four plates. Divide tofu mixture among lettuce leaves and serve hot.

Warm Chickpea Salad with Spinach

SERVES 4	
Calories	197
Fat	7g
Sodium	697mg
Carbohydrates	25g
Fiber	8g
Sugar	6g
Protein	9g

THE VERSATILE CHICKPEA

Chickpeas, also known as garbanzo beans, are a type of legume best known as the main ingredient in hummus. They are an excellent plant-based source of protein and have a high fiber content. Chickpeas are great for adding to salads or soups, and you can even whip the liquid from the can—called aquafaba—to create an egg substitute that can be used for baking desserts.

The key to staying energized is consuming as much of a variety of nutrients as possible. In under 15 minutes, you can enjoy this light protein-rich dish that nourishes your body.

1 tablespoon extra-virgin olive oil

4 cloves garlic, peeled and minced

1/2 medium yellow onion, peeled and diced

2 cups baby spinach

1 (15-ounce) can chickpeas, drained and rinsed

1/2 teaspoon ground cumin

1/2 teaspoon salt

1/8 teaspoon curry powder

1 1/2 tablespoons lemon juice

1/4 cup vegetable broth

1 Heat oil in a large skillet over medium-low heat. Sauté garlic and onion until translucent, about 5 minutes.

2 Stir in spinach, chickpeas, cumin, salt, and curry powder. Cook, stirring, for 2 minutes. Add lemon juice and broth and cook, stirring occasionally, until thoroughly heated, about 3 minutes.

Spinach and Tomato Tofu Scramble

Mashed tofu is a great substitute for scrambled eggs—it has a similar texture and consistency, and it's just as filling. Feel free to add your favorite toppings and make this dish your own.

8 ounces extra-firm tofu, drained, pressed, and cubed

1 tablespoon olive oil

2 cloves garlic, peeled and minced

1/2 cup chopped yellow onion

1 1/4 cups sliced button mushrooms

2 cups baby spinach

1/2 cup quartered cherry tomatoes

1/2 teaspoon ground turmeric

1/4 teaspoon salt

1/2 teaspoon ground black pepper

SERVES 2	
Calories	208
Fat	13g
Sodium	330mg
Carbohydrates	12g
Fiber	3g
Sugar	4g
Protein	15g

1 Place tofu in a medium bowl. Break up with a fork until crumbled. Set aside.

2 Heat oil in a medium skillet over medium-low heat. Add garlic and cook 1 minute, stirring frequently. Add onion and mushrooms; cook 4–5 minutes until onions are translucent and mushrooms begin to soften, stirring occasionally. Add spinach and cook about 2 minutes or until spinach begins to wilt.

3 Add tofu, tomatoes, and turmeric; sauté about 1 minute until tofu is heated through and all ingredients are evenly mixed. Season with salt and pepper. Serve warm.

Slow Cooker Tofu Scramble

SERVES 4	
Calories	124
Fat	10g
Sodium	299mg
Carbohydrates	1g
Fiber	0g
Sugar	1g
Protein	7g

This delicious protein scramble is perfect for breakfast or lunch. It also keeps for 3–4 days in the refrigerator, so you can cook it once and enjoy it later in the week.

2 tablespoons olive oil

1 (14-ounce) package firm tofu, drained, pressed and crumbled

2 cloves garlic, peeled and minced

1 teaspoon ground turmeric

1/2 teaspoon salt

1/4 teaspoon ground black pepper

3 tablespoons lemon juice

1/4 cup chopped fresh chives

1 Grease the bottom of a 4-quart slow cooker with oil. Add tofu, garlic, turmeric, salt, and pepper. Mix well. Cover and cook on low heat for 3 hours.

2 About 3 minutes before the scramble is fully cooked, stir in lemon juice. Sprinkle with chives before serving.

Vegetarian "Egg" Scramble

You can throw together this scramble for breakfast, lunch, or dinner in under 10 minutes. Extra soy milk will add a punch of protein on top of the tofu and nutritional yeast.

1 (12.3-ounce) package extra-firm tofu, drained, pressed, and cubed

1 teaspoon ground turmeric

1 teaspoon dried dill

¼ teaspoon garlic powder

1 teaspoon salt

½ teaspoon ground black pepper

2 tablespoons nutritional yeast

1 teaspoon minced fresh ginger

2 tablespoons minced yellow onion

1 tablespoon vegetable oil

2 tablespoons soy milk

1 Place tofu cubes in a medium bowl and use your fingers to crumble and break them up until tofu has the texture of scrambled egg.

2 Stir in turmeric, dill, garlic powder, salt, pepper, nutritional yeast, ginger, and onion.

3 Heat oil in a large skillet over medium-high heat. Add tofu mixture. Cook, stirring continually, for 2 minutes, then stir in soy milk.

4 Continue sautéing for 2 minutes or until tofu has a light, fluffy texture. Serve immediately.

SERVES 4	
Calories	117
Fat	8g
Sodium	585mg
Carbohydrates	2g
Fiber	1g
Sugar	0g
Protein	9g

WHAT IS NUTRITIONAL YEAST?

Nutritional yeast is a vegan and gluten-free seasoning with a slightly cheesy, umami flavor. It's made from baker's yeast that is cooked to deactivate the yeast and enhance its flavors, then crushed into a powder for use on food. Nutritional yeast is rich in protein, fiber, and B vitamins, and it contains no sodium, unlike other seasonings.

Egg Salad Sandwiches with Radish and Cilantro

SERVES 4	
Calories	195
Fat	11g
Sodium	238mg
Carbohydrates	12g
Fiber	3g
Sugar	2g
Protein	12g

If you have more flexibility and tolerance with your carbohydrate intake, try this tasty, crunchy sandwich. Add another slice of bread to top each sandwich if you like.

6 large eggs

1 cup shredded radish

¼ cup chopped fresh cilantro

1 tablespoon olive oil

1 tablespoon rice wine vinegar

¼ teaspoon ground black pepper

4 (1-ounce) slices low-carb bread

2 cups mixed baby greens

1 Place eggs in a medium saucepan and add enough water to cover by 1"–2". Place pan over high heat and bring to a boil. Reduce heat to medium-low and simmer for 12 minutes. Remove from heat and place under cold running water. When eggs are cool enough to handle, gently crack, peel, and dice. Place in a medium bowl.

2 Add radish, cilantro, oil, vinegar, and pepper and stir well to combine.

3 Place bread on four serving plates. Divide greens and egg mixture evenly among bread slices. Serve immediately.

CHAPTER 9

Snacks

Air-Fried Crispy Chickpeas

Craving a little spice and a little crunch? These low-glycemic nuggets are perfect for an on-the-go snack or a salad topping. Make a big batch so they're ready whenever you need a high-protein snack.

1 (15-ounce) can chickpeas, drained, rinsed, and patted dry

½ teaspoon salt

½ teaspoon chili powder

1 Preheat an air fryer to 400°F.
2 Place chickpeas in a large bowl. Spray with canola oil cooking spray and toss to coat evenly.
3 Place chickpeas in the air fryer basket and cook for 5 minutes. Stir chickpeas and cook for another 3 minutes.
4 Toss hot chickpeas with salt and chili powder. Cool for 5 minutes before serving.

SERVES 4	
Calories	155
Fat	3g
Sodium	638mg
Carbohydrates	23g
Fiber	8g
Sugar	5g
Protein	9g

SHOULD YOU USE CANNED OR DRIED CHICKPEAS?

The choice between canned and dried chickpeas depends on your needs: If you want convenience and speed, canned is the way to go. If you prefer cost-effectiveness and flavor control, dried chick-peas are ideal. Both are nutritious and versatile additions to any number of dishes!

Pepper Poppers

Traditional jalapeño poppers may be a little too spicy for you now. Mini sweet peppers make a safer choice for this party favorite.

6 mini sweet peppers, seeded and halved lengthwise

1 cup cream cheese, softened

1/2 teaspoon granulated garlic

1/2 teaspoon granulated onion

4 slices bacon, cooked and chopped

1/2 cup shredded pepper jack cheese

SERVES 6	
Calories	219
Fat	19g
Sodium	321mg
Carbohydrates	5g
Fiber	1g
Sugar	3g
Protein	7g

1 Preheat oven to 350°F. Line a large baking sheet with parchment paper.

2 Arrange peppers on the prepared baking sheet, cut side up.

3 Combine cream cheese, garlic, onion, and bacon in a medium bowl. Scoop 1 tablespoon cream cheese mixture into each pepper half.

4 Sprinkle cheese on top of stuffed peppers.

5 Bake for 20 minutes or until cheese is melted and peppers are slightly softened.

6 Remove from oven and allow to cool for 5 minutes before serving.

Spaghetti Squash Pizza Bites

SPAGHETTI MEETS SQUASH

To cook spaghetti squash in the microwave, poke holes into the squash using a fork, then microwave for 3–4 minutes. Remove the squash and cut it in half, scooping out the seeds. Put the halves into a microwave-safe dish, cut side down, and add 1" of water. Microwave for 5 minutes, then use a fork to scrape out the strands.

Enjoy the best parts of spaghetti and pizza without all the carbohydrates. If your appetite is low, use this as a small meal to graze on throughout the day.

1¼ cups cooked spaghetti squash "noodles"

1 large egg, beaten

½ cup pizza sauce

½ cup chopped pepperoni

½ cup shredded mozzarella cheese

12 fresh basil leaves

1. Preheat oven to 400°F. Grease a muffin pan with olive oil cooking spray.
2. Combine spaghetti squash, egg, and pizza sauce in a medium bowl and mix well. Scoop equal amounts of squash mixture into each muffin cup. Sprinkle with pepperoni and cheese and place a basil leaf on top of each.
3. Bake for 25 minutes or until set.
4. Remove from oven and allow to cool for 5 minutes before serving.

Salted Kale Chips

Salty and crunchy, kale chips are a satisfying low-carb alternative to potato chips. Kale is high in fiber and antioxidants, and it has a low glycemic index, which keeps blood sugar levels steady.

1 large bunch curly kale, stems removed and torn into bite-sized pieces

2 tablespoons olive oil

1 teaspoon coarse salt

1 Preheat oven to 350°F. Line 2 large baking sheets with parchment paper.

2 Put kale in a large bowl and drizzle with oil. Massage kale until evenly coated. Add more oil if needed to coat all pieces evenly.

3 Spread kale pieces in a single layer on baking sheets and sprinkle with salt.

4 Bake for 16 minutes, rotating pans after first 8 minutes. Bake until crispy but not burning. Serve immediately.

SERVES 4	
Calories	38
Fat	3g
Sodium	370mg
Carbohydrates	2g
Fiber	2g
Sugar	1g
Protein	1g

THE BODY'S NATURAL WARRIORS

Antioxidants are substances that protect your cells from damage caused by harmful molecules known as free radicals. These free radicals can damage cells and increase inflammation. Antioxidants neutralize free radicals, reducing their harmful effects. They are abundant in many fruits and vegetables, with berries boasting some of the highest antioxidant content.

Cheese and Veggie–Stuffed Artichokes

GREEK YOGURT VS. REGULAR YOGURT

Greek yogurt is thicker and creamier than regular yogurt, with a tangier flavor. This difference is due to the additional straining process, which also results in higher protein content and lower sugar levels. Many people who are lactose intolerant can enjoy Greek yogurt, as much of the lactose is removed during straining.

Need a dish for a dinner party? This elevated artichoke dish will impress your friends while also keeping you on track with your weight loss goals. Artichokes are rich in fiber, antioxidants, and other disease-fighting nutrients.

1 cup shredded Havarti cheese

2 tablespoons grated Parmesan cheese

1/4 cup plain low-fat yogurt

1/4 cup mayonnaise

1 tablespoon lemon juice

2 scallions, trimmed and chopped

1 tablespoon capers

1 cup grated carrot

1 cup quartered grape tomatoes

1/8 teaspoon salt

4 large globe artichokes

1 medium lemon, cut into wedges

1 In medium bowl, combine cheeses, yogurt, mayonnaise, lemon juice, scallions, and capers and mix well. Stir in carrot, tomatoes, and salt, and set aside.

2 Cut off the top inch of each artichoke. Cut off the sharp tip of each leaf. Pull off the tough outer leaves and discard. Rub cut edges with lemon wedges. Cut artichokes in half lengthwise.

3 Bring a large pot of salted water to a boil and add lemon wedges. Add artichokes and simmer for 20–25 minutes or until a leaf pulls easily from the artichoke. Cool, then carefully remove chokes with a spoon. Stuff artichokes with the cheese mixture.

4 Preheat broiler. Place artichokes on a large ungreased baking sheet and broil for 3 minutes before serving.

Cheese Coins

These little crackers are excellent served warm with soup.
They also make a great addition to a tray with crudités.

SERVES 8	
Calories	374
Fat	24g
Sodium	574mg
Carbohydrates	24g
Fiber	1g
Sugar	0g
Protein	16g

$1/4$ cup butter

$1^{1}/2$ cups shredded sharp Cheddar cheese

$2/3$ cup shredded part-skim mozzarella cheese

1 tablespoon yellow mustard

2 tablespoons 1% milk

$1/2$ teaspoon seasoned salt

$1^{1}/2$ cups all-purpose flour

$1/4$ cup shredded Parmesan cheese

1 In a large bowl, combine butter with Cheddar, mozzarella, mustard, milk, and salt; beat until combined. Add flour and mix just until a dough forms.

2 Preheat oven to 350°F.

3 Shape dough into ½" balls and place on ungreased baking sheets. Press each ball with the bottom of a drinking glass to flatten to ⅛" thick. Sprinkle with Parmesan.

4 Bake crackers until light golden brown around edges, about 12–15 minutes. Remove from baking sheets and let cool completely on a wire rack. Store in airtight container at room temperature for up to one week.

Low-Carb Prosciutto Cup

SERVES 1	
Calories	198
Fat	15g
Sodium	644mg
Carbohydrates	2g
Fiber	0g
Sugar	0g
Protein	14g

If you're craving pizza but can't tolerate it anymore, this low-carb cup will hit the spot. Stick to the serving size since the sodium count is high.

1 (0.5-ounce) slice prosciutto

1 medium egg yolk

½ ounce diced Brie cheese

½ ounce grated Parmesan cheese

½ teaspoon sriracha sauce (optional)

1 Preheat oven to 350°F. Use a muffin pan with cups about 2½" wide and 1½" deep.
2 Fold prosciutto slice in half so it becomes almost square. Place it in a muffin pan cup to line it completely. Top with egg yolk.
3 Sprinkle with cheeses and drizzle with sriracha.
4 Bake for 12 minutes or until yolk is cooked and warm but still runny. Let cool for 10 minutes before removing from muffin pan.

Pepperoni Cheese Bites

SERVES 2	
Calories	240
Fat	19g
Sodium	647mg
Carbohydrates	2g
Fiber	0g
Sugar	1g
Protein	15g

With just two ingredients and zero prep time, this snack is an easy option for quick calories and protein. Enjoy them cold or warm them in a toaster oven just until the cheese melts for a warm, tasty treat.

4 (1-ounce) sticks mozzarella string cheese

16 slices sugar-free pepperoni

1 Cut each string cheese stick lengthwise into four equal pieces.
2 Wrap each piece in a slice of pepperoni and secure with a toothpick. Serve immediately.

Sweet and Sour Sauce

For a fun and healthy snack, dip small chunks of cooked chicken and steamed broccoli into this flavorful sauce. It's also great with Air-Fried Tofu (see recipe in Chapter 8).

2½ ounces pineapple juice

2½ tablespoons maple syrup

1 tablespoon plus 2 teaspoons rice vinegar

1¼ teaspoons tomato paste

2 teaspoons coconut aminos

1¼ teaspoons arrowroot powder

2 teaspoons warm water

SERVES 5	
Calories	38
Fat	0g
Sodium	36mg
Carbohydrates	9g
Fiber	0g
Sugar	8g
Protein	0g

1 In a small saucepan, whisk together pineapple juice, maple syrup, rice vinegar, tomato paste, and coconut aminos. Bring to a gentle simmer over medium heat. Remove from heat.

2 In a small bowl, combine arrowroot powder and water until smooth. Add the mixture to the saucepan and whisk for about 30 seconds to thicken.

3 Set aside to cool completely and transfer to an airtight container or serve immediately. Sauce will keep in the refrigerator for up to one week.

Stuffed Avocados

Avocados are nutrient dense and rich in monounsaturated fats and fiber, so the net carbohydrates are low. When making this recipe, choose an avocado that is ripe but still firm. If the avocado is too soft, it'll be too mushy and won't hold the tuna as well.

SERVES 2	
Calories	239
Fat	20g
Sodium	232mg
Carbohydrates	6g
Fiber	5g
Sugar	1g
Protein	9g

READY TO DITCH THE MAYO?

If you're looking for a healthier alternative to mayonnaise, the closest in terms of texture and taste is Greek yogurt or sour cream. You can also experiment with hummus, mashed avocado, whipped cottage cheese, or even silken tofu.

1 large avocado

1 (5-ounce) can water-packed light tuna, drained

2 tablespoons mayonnaise

1/2 medium green bell pepper, seeded and chopped

1/4 teaspoon dried minced onion

1/8 teaspoon garlic salt

1/8 teaspoon ground black pepper

1 Cut avocado in half lengthwise and remove the pit. Set aside.

2 In a medium mixing bowl, combine tuna, mayonnaise, bell pepper, onion, garlic salt, and black pepper and mash together with a fork.

3 Scoop half of the mixture into each avocado half. Serve.

Air Fryer Greek Deviled Eggs

Did you know you could make hard-cooked eggs in an air fryer? Make some extra eggs to keep in the refrigerator for an easy snack throughout the week.

4 large eggs

2 tablespoons plain low-fat Greek yogurt

2 tablespoons pitted and finely chopped Kalamata olives

2 tablespoons goat cheese crumbles

⅛ teaspoon salt

⅛ teaspoon freshly ground black pepper

2 tablespoons minced fresh mint

1 Preheat air fryer to 250°F.

2 Place eggs in individual silicone muffin cups. Add silicone cups to the air fryer basket. Cook for 15 minutes.

3 Fill a medium bowl with cold water and ice. Transfer eggs to the water bath immediately to stop cooking process. After 5 minutes, remove and carefully peel eggs.

4 Cut eggs in half lengthwise. Spoon yolks into a separate medium bowl. Arrange white halves on a large plate.

5 Using a fork, blend egg yolks with yogurt, olives, goat cheese, salt, and pepper. Spoon mixture into white halves. Garnish with mint and serve.

SERVES 4	
Calories	89
Fat	6g
Sodium	179mg
Carbohydrates	1g
Fiber	0g
Sugar	0g
Protein	8g

DEVILED EGG DOS AND DON'TS

Deviled eggs are a perfect high-protein treat that you can prepare ahead of time. To achieve a super smooth filling, press the yolks through a sieve to eliminate any clumps. To avoid the mess of filling the egg whites, skip the spoon and use the snipped corner of a plastic storage bag to pipe in the filling.

Ham and Egg Cups

SERVES 6	
Calories	248
Fat	19g
Sodium	734mg
Carbohydrates	1g
Fiber	0g
Sugar	0g
Protein	18g

Make these cups on a Sunday night and keep them in the refrigerator for a quick breakfast, snack, or even small lunch during the week. The cups can also be individually wrapped and frozen.

8 large eggs, beaten

1/4 cup heavy cream

1/4 teaspoon garlic powder

1/2 teaspoon salt

1/4 teaspoon ground black pepper

1 cup grated Cheddar cheese

2 cups baby spinach

6 (1-ounce) slices deli ham

2 tablespoons chopped fresh chives

1 Preheat oven to 375°F. Spray a 6-cup large muffin pan with nonstick cooking spray or line the cups with paper liners. Set aside.

2 Combine eggs, cream, garlic powder, salt, and pepper in a medium mixing bowl. Whisk until well combined. Stir in cheese and spinach.

3 Line each muffin cup with a slice of ham. Fill each cup with an equal amount of egg mixture.

4 Bake for 25 minutes until eggs are set. Garnish with chives and serve immediately.

Horseradish, Turkey, Swiss, and Bacon Cups

If you're looking for a low-carb snack with a kick, this is the recipe for you! These little cups are crunchy, cheesy, and salty, with a bright little kiss of heat from the horseradish.

3 tablespoons Dijon mustard

1¹/₂ teaspoons prepared horseradish

6 (1-ounce) slices deli turkey

6 (1-ounce) slices Swiss cheese

1 cup halved cherry tomatoes

2 large Bibb lettuce leaves, roughly chopped

2 pieces cooked bacon, crumbled

SERVES 6	
Calories	165
Fat	10g
Sodium	302mg
Carbohydrates	2g
Fiber	0g
Sugar	1g
Protein	17g

1 Preheat oven to 375°F.

2 In a small bowl, whisk together mustard and horseradish. Set aside.

3 Line the cups of a nonstick, 6-cup large muffin pan with turkey slices. Top with cheese slices. Bake for 8–10 minutes until turkey is lightly crisped and cheese is melted.

4 Using an offset spatula, divide mustard mixture between the cups. Top with tomatoes, lettuce, and bacon. Serve immediately.

Low-Carb Turkey Pesto Wrap

SERVES 4	
Calories	329
Fat	18g
Sodium	894mg
Carbohydrates	26g
Fiber	17g
Sugar	2g
Protein	16g

A jar of prepared pesto in your refrigerator can be your secret weapon when you need to add calories to a meal. It's full of healthy, anti-inflammatory fats. Spread it on sandwiches or wraps, stir it into soup, or use it as a sauce for some high-protein pasta.

¼ **cup pesto sauce**

4 (6") low-carb soft tortillas

8 (1-ounce) slices deli roasted turkey

1 medium avocado, peeled, pitted, and sliced

1½ cups salad greens

1 Spread 1 tablespoon pesto on each tortilla. Layer 2 slices turkey, ¼ of the avocado, and lettuce on top of pesto.

2 Roll tortillas around fillings and serve.

Yogurt and Almond Butter Dip

SERVES 4	
Calories	143
Fat	8g
Sodium	12mg
Carbohydrates	11g
Fiber	2g
Sugar	8g
Protein	7g

This tasty and healthy dip pairs wonderfully with fruit or can be used as a spread on crackers or toast.

½ **cup plain low-fat Greek yogurt**

¼ **cup unsalted almond butter**

2 tablespoons maple syrup

Combine all ingredients in a small bowl. Mix until smooth. Serve at room temperature or refrigerate for 1–2 hours.

Cottage Cheese Fall Salad

This protein-packed snack is full of warm fall flavors. Try whipping the cottage cheese in a food processor if you like a creamier consistency.

2 cups low-fat cottage cheese

1 teaspoon ground cinnamon

1/2 teaspoon ground nutmeg

1 large red apple, cored and thinly sliced

2 tablespoons apple juice

1/2 teaspoon salt

1/4 teaspoon ground black pepper

SERVES 4	
Calories	162
Fat	3g
Sodium	561mg
Carbohydrates	15g
Fiber	1g
Sugar	12g
Protein	18g

Combine all ingredients in a medium mixing bowl. Cover bowl with plastic wrap and refrigerate until ready to serve.

Fruit and Cheese Kebabs

Berries are a good choice for snacking because they contain fructose, a natural sugar that doesn't require insulin to be metabolized. And the fiber in berries helps slow down the absorption of sugar into the bloodstream.

4 (1-ounce) slices Cheddar cheese

10 medium strawberries, hulled

10 blueberries

SERVES 2	
Calories	296
Fat	19g
Sodium	407mg
Carbohydrates	17g
Fiber	4g
Sugar	13g
Protein	14g

1 Cut Cheddar into fun shapes like stars or hearts with 1" cookie cutters. You will use 2 cheese slices for each skewer.
2 Thread fruit and cheese onto wooden skewers: first a strawberry, then a blueberry, then a piece of cheese, and so on—alternate to create a pattern.
3 Serve immediately or place in a flat storage container and refrigerate overnight.

Bacon and Sun-Dried Tomato Dip

Pair this sizzling dip with celery and carrot sticks or bell pepper wedges for a low-carb appetizer or snack. If regular pork bacon is too heavy for you, use turkey bacon instead.

SERVES 6	
Calories	199
Fat	15g
Sodium	354mg
Carbohydrates	2g
Fiber	0g
Sugar	1g
Protein	14g

1 (15-ounce) container whole milk ricotta cheese

¼ cup shredded Parmesan cheese

¼ cup shredded mozzarella cheese

2 tablespoons chopped sun-dried tomatoes

6 slices bacon, cooked and chopped

¼ teaspoon crushed red pepper flakes

1 Preheat oven to 375°F.

2 Combine all ingredients in a large mixing bowl and stir until incorporated. Transfer to an ungreased 8" × 8" baking dish and bake for 20 minutes or until bubbly and golden brown.

3 Remove from oven and allow to cool.

4 Divide into six equal portions and transfer each portion to a separate airtight container. Store in the refrigerator until ready to eat, up to one week.

GET GREAT AT CHEESE GRATING

Pre-grated cheese often contains anti-caking agents that can affect melting and flavor, so grating fresh cheese is usually the better option, even if it's a bit of a hassle. Place softer cheeses in the freezer for 30 minutes before grating. For harder cheeses, be sure to grate against the grain for a more even consistency.

CHAPTER 10

Dessert

Black Bean Brownies

SERVES 12

Calories	141
Fat	6g
Sodium	53mg
Carbohydrates	18g
Fiber	3g
Sugar	13g
Protein	3g

ARE THEY READY?

To determine if brownies are ready to come out of the oven, look for a few key indicators. Insert a toothpick or thin knife into the center; if it comes out with a few moist crumbs, they're done. Gently touch the top layer—if it feels very soft or jiggly, they need more time.

Don't worry—you can't taste the beans in these fudgy brownies. This secret ingredient adds the perfect moisture and texture to these brownies, along with a boost of protein and fiber.

¼ cup plus 1 teaspoon melted coconut oil, divided

3 tablespoons warm water

2 tablespoons ground flaxseed

1 (15-ounce) can unsalted black beans, drained and rinsed

¼ cup almond flour

¼ cup unsweetened cocoa powder

½ cup coconut sugar

1 teaspoon vanilla extract

¼ teaspoon salt

1 teaspoon baking powder

¼ cup semisweet chocolate chips

1 Preheat oven to 350°F. Grease an 8" × 8" baking dish with 1 teaspoon coconut oil.

2 Prepare the flaxseed "egg" by adding water and flaxseed to a small bowl. Stir and let sit for 15 minutes, until flaxseeds are gummy. Transfer to a blender or food processor.

3 Add remaining ¼ cup coconut oil, beans, flour, cocoa, sugar, vanilla, salt, and baking powder, and blend on high until the mixture is smooth, about 1 minute. Stir in chocolate chips.

4 Spoon the batter evenly into the prepared pan. Bake for 20–30 minutes, until the outside begins to get crisp. Let cool for 15 minutes to set. Serve immediately or store in the refrigerator for up to one week.

Chocolate Mug Cake

A mug cake recipe is perfect when you need a sweet treat but only want one serving. You won't even be able to taste the pumpkin. It's just there to give a smooth, cake-like consistency to this quick, simple snack. This will be a recipe you make again and again!

2 large egg whites

1/4 cup pumpkin purée

2 tablespoons almond flour

1 tablespoon granulated stevia

1 tablespoon unsweetened cocoa powder

1/4 teaspoon baking powder

1/4 teaspoon vanilla extract

1/8 teaspoon salt

1 teaspoon unsweetened rice milk

1 Combine all ingredients in a microwave-safe mug. Stir to mix thoroughly.

2 Microwave for 2 minutes on high or until cake is set. Serve immediately.

SERVES 1	
Calories	155
Fat	6g
Sodium	403mg
Carbohydrates	13g
Fiber	2g
Sugar	1g
Protein	12g

MICROWAVING MADE EASY

There's not much you can't cook in the microwave if you use the right approach. To ensure even cooking, spread the food in a single layer and cut it into smaller pieces. For larger meals, remember to stir or turn the food halfway through. Additionally, keep your microwave clean to prevent any food safety hazards.

Vanilla Mug Cake

SERVES 1	
Calories	140
Fat	9g
Sodium	80mg
Carbohydrates	6g
Fiber	3g
Sugar	1g
Protein	9g

All you need are five ingredients and a minute or so in the microwave to satisfy your sweet tooth! Using stevia instead of sugar will keep your blood sugar steady without compromising on flavor.

1 large egg

1 tablespoon coconut flour

1 tablespoon almond flour

1 teaspoon vanilla extract

2/3 teaspoon granulated stevia

1 Beat egg in a microwave-safe mug. Add remaining ingredients and whisk with a fork until combined.

2 Microwave for 60–90 seconds on high until cake is set. Allow to cool slightly before serving.

Mango Yogurt Pudding

SERVES 4	
Calories	151
Fat	6g
Sodium	55mg
Carbohydrates	11g
Fiber	1g
Sugar	9g
Protein	14g

For optimal blood sugar balance, pair carbohydrate-rich foods like mangoes with high-protein ingredients to buffer the blood sugar response.

2 cups plain full-fat Greek yogurt

1/2 cup canned mango, finely chopped

2 tablespoons vanilla protein powder

1 Place all ingredients in a bowl and mix well.

2 Cover and refrigerate for about 30 minutes before serving.

Grilled Peach "Cobbler" Parfaits

These parfaits are light, individual desserts that you can enjoy, even with a smaller appetite. Grilling the peaches caramelizes the sugar on the outside. Top the parfaits off with a generous sprinkling of cinnamon for extra blood sugar–balancing benefits.

4 medium peaches, pitted and quartered

2 cups plain low-fat Greek yogurt

1 tablespoon honey

1 teaspoon ground cinnamon

6 shortbread cookies, crumbled

1 Preheat a gas or charcoal grill to medium heat.

2 Grill peaches until just browned, 1–2 minutes on each side. Remove peaches from grill and set aside to cool slightly, then slice each quarter into 2 or 3 slices.

3 Combine yogurt, honey, and cinnamon in a medium bowl.

4 In six small glasses or cups, layer a dollop of yogurt, a few peach slices, and 2 teaspoons cookie crumbs. Repeat layering one more time, ending with cookie crumbs on top. Serve immediately.

SERVES 6	
Calories	247
Fat	10g
Sodium	133mg
Carbohydrates	30g
Fiber	2g
Sugar	18g
Protein	9g

CINNAMON AND YOUR CELLS

Cinnamon helps lower blood sugar levels by improving insulin sensitivity, allowing cells to use glucose more efficiently. It can also slow the breakdown of carbohydrates in the digestive system, leading to more stable blood sugar levels after meals. Due to its reputation for managing blood sugar, cinnamon is available in supplement form as well.

Berry Protein Yogurt Delight

SERVES 4	
Calories	173
Fat	11g
Sodium	114mg
Carbohydrates	12g
Fiber	3g
Sugar	2g
Protein	6g

Mixing whipped cream with yogurt gives it a creamy texture, and the raspberry swirl adds the perfect pop of flavor. This delightful dessert can be made with any fresh or frozen berries—try strawberry, blackberry, or blueberry.

1/2 cup fresh or frozen raspberries

1 teaspoon honey

1/2 teaspoon lemon juice

1 1/2 cups plain nonfat Greek yogurt

3 tablespoons vanilla protein powder, divided

1/4 cup heavy cream

1 Combine raspberries, honey, and lemon juice in a small microwave-safe bowl. Microwave on high for 2 minutes. Press through a fine mesh sieve into a small bowl to remove seeds. Cool for 30 minutes and refrigerate until needed.

2 Combine yogurt and 2 tablespoons protein powder in a medium bowl. Chill in refrigerator while you whip cream.

3 In a separate medium bowl, whip cream until moderately stiff; stir in the remaining 1 tablespoon protein powder.

4 Gently fold cream into yogurt mixture. Spoon mixture into four dessert or parfait cups. Swirl 1 tablespoon prepared raspberry sauce into each cup and serve.

Pumpkin Blondies

Here's a healthier twist for all the pumpkin spice lovers out there! Using almond flour and stevia in place of wheat flour and sugar cuts down on the carbohydrates in each brownie. Puréed pumpkin adds not only a lovely fall flavor but also several beneficial nutrients, like vitamin A.

2 cups almond flour

$1/2$ cup ground flaxseed

1 tablespoon granulated stevia

$1/2$ teaspoon salt

2 teaspoons almond extract

1 cup pumpkin purée

1 large egg

1 Preheat oven to 350°F. Grease an 8" × 8" baking dish.

2 In a medium mixing bowl, combine almond flour, flaxseed, stevia, and salt.

3 In a large bowl, mix almond extract, pumpkin purée, and egg until combined.

4 Fold dry ingredients into wet ingredients until just combined. Do not overmix. Pour mixture into the prepared pan.

5 Bake for 20–25 minutes, until blondies are set and a toothpick inserted in the center comes out clean.

SERVES 12	
Calories	163
Fat	11g
Sodium	104mg
Carbohydrates	10g
Fiber	4g
Sugar	1g
Protein	6g

WHAT IS STEVIA?

Stevia is a natural, plant-based sweetener that has almost no calories and is much sweeter than table sugar. Best of all, it has no impact on blood sugar! Stevia is available in powder form, which is ideal for baking, and as liquid drops, which work well in smoothies and puddings.

Cookie Dough Energy Bites

SERVES 8	
Calories	241
Fat	17g
Sodium	15mg
Carbohydrates	14g
Fiber	5g
Sugar	8g
Protein	8g

SUBSTITUTING DATES

Dates have been cultivated for thousands of years and are a staple in Middle Eastern cuisine. With a low glycemic index, they don't cause a large spike in blood sugar, making them a healthier alternative to regular table sugar. Dates are often puréed into a paste and used as a sweetener and binder in raw treats and baked goods.

If the GLP-1 medication is causing you to feel fatigued, try this fun pick-me-up. The dates and cacao add a dose of sweetness while the almond butter evens out the flavors and the macronutrient profile.

½ cup creamy almond butter

½ cup hemp hearts

½ cup coconut flakes

8 large dates, pitted

1 teaspoon vanilla extract

¼ cup cacao nibs

¼ cup raw cacao powder

1 In a food processor or high-speed blender, pulse together almond butter, hemp, coconut, dates, and vanilla until a thick dough forms. Fold in cacao nibs. Roll into 1" balls and dust with cacao powder.

2 Store bites in refrigerator. Enjoy within three weeks.

Low-Carb Lemon Custard

Have your cake and eat it too with this carb-conscious dessert. Lemons contain a natural compound called hesperidin that may lower blood sugar levels.

1/4 cup butter

2 ounces cream cheese

2 tablespoons lemon juice

2 teaspoons grated lemon zest

10 drops liquid stevia

4 large egg yolks

1/8 teaspoon xanthan gum

SERVES 2	
Calories	414
Fat	42g
Sodium	288mg
Carbohydrates	2g
Fiber	0g
Sugar	1g
Protein	7g

1 Melt butter and cream cheese in a small saucepan over medium-low heat, about 2 minutes. Add lemon juice, lemon zest, and stevia, stirring constantly until the mixture comes together.

2 Slowly add in one egg yolk at a time, constantly whisking, until the mixture is smooth and creamy. Allow to cook for an additional 2–3 minutes, then add in xanthan gum and stir until combined.

3 Remove from heat and pour the mixture into a bowl. Cover the custard with plastic wrap, pressing onto the surface. Refrigerate for at least 2 hours before serving.

Mocha Mini Soufflés

Impress your family and friends with this harmonious chocolate and coffee combination. Whipping in extra egg whites adds a fluffy texture and extra protein at the same time.

WHIPPING EGG WHITES RIGHT

When whipping egg whites, it's essential to use a right-sized bowl. It should provide enough room for the whites to expand without being so large that they spread too thin. Ensure your bowl is spotlessly clean, as any residue of fat can prevent the egg whites from stiffening properly.

3 tablespoons butter

1½ tablespoons all-purpose flour

1 tablespoon natural cocoa powder

1 tablespoon instant espresso powder

⅛ teaspoon salt

¾ cup whole milk, room temperature

4 ounces bittersweet chocolate, finely chopped

4 large egg yolks, room temperature

1 teaspoon vanilla extract

6 large egg whites, room temperature

⅓ cup superfine sugar

¼ cup confectioners' sugar

1 Preheat oven to 400°F. Butter six individual soufflé dishes. Set aside.

2 Melt 3 tablespoons butter in a heavy-bottomed saucepan over medium heat. Whisk in flour, cocoa powder, espresso powder, and salt until thickened (about 2 minutes). Slowly add milk and bring to a boil, whisking continuously. Remove from the heat and whisk in chocolate until smooth. Whisk in egg yolks, one at a time, and vanilla. Set aside.

3 Whip egg whites, using an electric mixer on a high speed, until soft peaks form. Sprinkle in superfine sugar and beat until stiff peaks begin to form. Fold a quarter of egg whites into the chocolate mixture. Lightly fold in the remaining egg whites.

4 Pour into the prepared dishes. Place dishes on a large baking sheet and bake for 15 minutes or until puffed. The soufflés should be baked around the outside edges and creamy in the centers.

5 Dust with sifted confectioners' sugar and serve warm.

Vegan Lemon-Infused Olive Oil Ice Cream

Tofu in ice cream? Don't count this recipe out until you've tried it! The unexpected combination of tofu, olive oil, and coconut will pleasantly surprise you with a rich, smooth texture and keep your blood sugar happy.

12 ounces extra-firm tofu, drained

½ cup extra-virgin olive oil

½ cup canned coconut milk

2 teaspoons grated lemon zest

⅛ teaspoon salt

¼ cup maple syrup

SERVES 8	
Calories	202
Fat	17g
Sodium	42mg
Carbohydrates	8g
Fiber	1g
Sugar	7g
Protein	4g

1 Blend all ingredients in a blender until smooth. Refrigerate for 4 hours or overnight.

2 Add mixture to an ice cream maker and follow manufacturer's instructions for freezing.

Chunky Monkey Mocha Shake

SERVES 1	
Calories	357
Fat	3g
Sodium	86mg
Carbohydrates	60g
Fiber	7g
Sugar	37g
Protein	22g

GREEN BANANAS: RESISTANT STARCH

Green bananas contain resistant starch, a polysaccharide with many potential health benefits. Resistant starch can help to increase metabolism, lower blood sugar levels, reduce cholesterol levels, and help prevent diabetes. It's also a prebiotic fiber that can help boost the immune system. So when choosing bananas, go green!

What a delicious treat for a hot day! The Fairlife milk and protein powder add an extra boost of protein. Frozen bananas provide a smooth and creamy texture.

2 large bananas, peeled, sliced, and frozen

1/2 cup 2% Fairlife Ultra-Filtered Milk

1 tablespoon chocolate protein powder

1 teaspoon instant coffee granules

1 tablespoon whipped cream

2 teaspoons sugar-free chocolate syrup

1 Place bananas, milk, protein powder, and coffee in a blender and blend until smooth.

2 Pour into a tall glass and top with whipped cream and a drizzle of chocolate syrup. Serve immediately.

APPENDIX A

Meal Plans

If your schedule is better suited to eating three substantial meals per day, this meal plan provides an example of how to meet all of your calorie and macronutrient goals.

	Breakfast	Lunch
Meal Plan Week 1: Full Meals		
Monday	Soft Scrambled Eggs on Toast ➤ **Appendix B** Simple Vanilla Protein Shake ➤ **Appendix B**	Tangy Sirloin Salad ➤ **Chapter 6**
Tuesday	Soft Scrambled Eggs on Toast ➤ **Appendix B** Simple Vanilla Protein Shake ➤ **Appendix B**	Tangy Sirloin Salad ➤ **Chapter 6**
Wednesday	Soft Scrambled Eggs on Toast ➤ **Appendix B** Simple Vanilla Protein Shake ➤ **Appendix B**	Tangy Sirloin Salad ➤ **Chapter 6**
Thursday	Baked "Sausage" and Mushroom Frittata ➤ **Chapter 5** Cinnamon Smoothie ➤ **Chapter 5**	Tangy Sirloin Salad ➤ **Chapter 6**
Friday	Baked "Sausage" and Mushroom Frittata ➤ **Chapter 5** Cinnamon Smoothie ➤ **Chapter 5**	Quick Curry Chicken ➤ **Chapter 6**
Saturday	Baked "Sausage" and Mushroom Frittata ➤ **Chapter 5** Cinnamon Smoothie ➤ **Chapter 5**	Quick Curry Chicken ➤ **Chapter 6**
Sunday	Baked "Sausage" and Mushroom Frittata ➤ **Chapter 5** Cinnamon Smoothie ➤ **Chapter 5**	Quick Curry Chicken ➤ **Chapter 6**

Meal Plan Week 1: Full Meals—continued

	Dinner	Snack
Monday	Baked Red Snapper Veracruz ► Chapter 7	Mango Yogurt Pudding ► Chapter 10
Tuesday	Baked Red Snapper Veracruz ► Chapter 7	Mango Yogurt Pudding ► Chapter 10
Wednesday	Baked Red Snapper Veracruz ► Chapter 7	Mango Yogurt Pudding ► Chapter 10
Thursday	Instant Pot® Italian Beef and Peppers ► Chapter 6	Mango Yogurt Pudding ► Chapter 10
Friday	Instant Pot® Italian Beef and Peppers ► Chapter 6	
Saturday	Instant Pot® Italian Beef and Peppers ► Chapter 6	
Sunday	Instant Pot® Italian Beef and Peppers ► Chapter 6	

Meal Plan Week 2: Full Meals

	Breakfast	Lunch
Monday	Berry Protein Yogurt Delight ➤ Chapter 10 Perfect Poached Eggs on Toast ➤ Chapter 5	Instant Pot® Turmeric Chicken and Cabbage Soup ➤ Chapter 6
Tuesday	Berry Protein Yogurt Delight ➤ Chapter 10 Perfect Poached Eggs on Toast ➤ Chapter 5	Instant Pot® Turmeric Chicken and Cabbage Soup ➤ Chapter 6
Wednesday	Berry Protein Yogurt Delight ➤ Chapter 10 Perfect Poached Eggs on Toast ➤ Chapter 5	Instant Pot® Turmeric Chicken and Cabbage Soup ➤ Chapter 6
Thursday	Huevos Rancheros Breakfast Casserole ➤ Chapter 5 Simple Vanilla Protein Shake ➤ Appendix B	Instant Pot® Turmeric Chicken and Cabbage Soup ➤ Chapter 6
Friday	Huevos Rancheros Breakfast Casserole ➤ Chapter 5 Simple Vanilla Protein Shake ➤ Appendix B	Avocado and Shrimp Salad ➤ Chapter 7
Saturday	Huevos Rancheros Breakfast Casserole ➤ Chapter 5 Simple Vanilla Protein Shake ➤ Appendix B	Avocado and Shrimp Salad ➤ Chapter 7
Sunday	Huevos Rancheros Breakfast Casserole ➤ Chapter 5 Simple Vanilla Protein Shake ➤ Appendix B	Chicken Mushroom Marinara Bake ➤ Chapter 6

	Dinner	Snack
Monday	Ancho-Rubbed Salmon with Avocado Salsa ➤ Chapter 7	
Tuesday	Ancho-Rubbed Salmon with Avocado Salsa ➤ Chapter 7	
Wednesday	Chicken Mushroom Marinara Bake ➤ Chapter 6	
Thursday	Chicken Mushroom Marinara Bake ➤ Chapter 6	Grilled Peach "Cobbler" Parfaits ➤ Chapter 10
Friday	Chicken Mushroom Marinara Bake ➤ Chapter 6	Grilled Peach "Cobbler" Parfaits ➤ Chapter 10
Saturday	Jumbo Sweet and Spicy Shrimp Skewers ➤ Chapter 7	Grilled Peach "Cobbler" Parfaits ➤ Chapter 10
Sunday	Jumbo Sweet and Spicy Shrimp Skewers ➤ Chapter 7	Grilled Peach "Cobbler" Parfaits ➤ Chapter 10

Meal Plan Week 2: Full Meals—continued

If you're experiencing stronger side effects or a reduced appetite, try a meal plan like this, which divides the calories and macros into six smaller meals throughout the day.

	Meal Plan Week 1: Small Meals		
	Breakfast	**Snack 1**	**Lunch**
Monday	Danish Egg Cake with Bacon and Tomatoes ➤ Chapter 5	Chicken and Vegetable Frittata ➤ Chapter 6	Lemon Dill Tuna Salad Lettuce Cups ➤ Chapter 7
Tuesday	Danish Egg Cake with Bacon and Tomatoes ➤ Chapter 5	Chicken and Vegetable Frittata ➤ Chapter 6	Lemon Dill Tuna Salad Lettuce Cups ➤ Chapter 7
Wednesday	Danish Egg Cake with Bacon and Tomatoes ➤ Chapter 5	Chicken and Vegetable Frittata ➤ Chapter 6	Lemon Dill Tuna Salad Lettuce Cups ➤ Chapter 7
Thursday	High-Protein Cottage Cheese Pancakes ➤ Chapter 5	Oil-Free Scrambled Egg Whites ➤ Appendix B 1 slice low-carb bread	Low-Carb Cabbage Wrap Street Tacos ➤ Chapter 6
Friday	High-Protein Cottage Cheese Pancakes ➤ Chapter 5	Oil-Free Scrambled Egg Whites ➤ Appendix B 1 slice low-carb bread	Lemon Dill Tuna Salad Lettuce Cups ➤ Chapter 7
Saturday	High-Protein Cottage Cheese Pancakes ➤ Chapter 5	Oil-Free Scrambled Egg Whites ➤ Appendix B 1 slice low-carb bread	Low-Carb Cabbage Wrap Street Tacos ➤ Chapter 6
Sunday	Chocolate Peanut Butter Smoothie ➤ Chapter 5	Oil-Free Scrambled Egg Whites ➤ Appendix B 1 slice low-carb bread	Low-Carb Cabbage Wrap Street Tacos ➤ Chapter 6

	Meal Plan Week 1: Small Meals—continued		
	Snack 2	**Dinner**	**Snack 3**
Monday	Cottage Cheese Fall Salad ► Chapter 9 Pepperoni Cheese Bites ► Chapter 9	Slow Cooker Chicken Chili Verde ► Chapter 6	Chocolate Mug Cake ► Chapter 10
Tuesday	Cottage Cheese Fall Salad ► Chapter 9 Pepperoni Cheese Bites ► Chapter 9	Slow Cooker Chicken Chili Verde ► Chapter 6	Chocolate Mug Cake ► Chapter 10
Wednesday	Cottage Cheese Fall Salad ► Chapter 9 Low-Carb Prosciutto Cup ► Chapter 9	Slow Cooker Chicken Chili Verde ► Chapter 6	Chocolate Mug Cake ► Chapter 10
Thursday	Cottage Cheese Fall Salad ► Chapter 9 Low-Carb Prosciutto Cup ► Chapter 9	Orange Beef and Broccolini Stir-Fry ► Chapter 6	Vanilla Mug Cake ► Chapter 10
Friday	Horseradish, Turkey, Swiss, and Bacon Cups ► Chapter 9 Salted Kale Chips ► Chapter 9	Orange Beef and Broccolini Stir-Fry ► Chapter 6	Vanilla Mug Cake ► Chapter 10
Saturday	Horseradish, Turkey, Swiss, and Bacon Cups ► Chapter 9 Salted Kale Chips ► Chapter 9	Orange Beef and Broccolini Stir-Fry ► Chapter 6	Vanilla Mug Cake ► Chapter 10
Sunday	Horseradish, Turkey, Swiss, and Bacon Cups ► Chapter 9 Salted Kale Chips ► Chapter 9	Instant Pot® Salmon with Lemon and Dill ► Chapter 7	Vanilla Mug Cake ► Chapter 10

Meal Plan Week 2: Small Meals

	Breakfast	Snack 1	Lunch
Monday	Berry Protein Yogurt Delight ➤ Chapter 10	"Sausage" Egg Cups ➤ Chapter 5	Pineapple Shrimp Fried Rice ➤ Chapter 7
Tuesday	Berry Protein Yogurt Delight ➤ Chapter 10	"Sausage" Egg Cups ➤ Chapter 5	Pineapple Shrimp Fried Rice ➤ Chapter 7
Wednesday	Berry Protein Yogurt Delight ➤ Chapter 10	"Sausage" Egg Cups ➤ Chapter 5	Pineapple Shrimp Fried Rice ➤ Chapter 7
Thursday	Berry Protein Yogurt Delight ➤ Chapter 10	"Sausage" Egg Cups ➤ Chapter 5	Kung Pao Chicken ➤ Chapter 6
Friday	Simple Chocolate Protein Shake ➤ Appendix B	Scrambled Eggs ➤ Appendix B	Basil, Eggplant, and Tofu Stir-Fry ➤ Chapter 8
Saturday	Simple Chocolate Protein Shake ➤ Appendix B	Scrambled Eggs ➤ Appendix B	Kung Pao Chicken ➤ Chapter 6
Sunday	Simple Chocolate Protein Shake ➤ Appendix B	Scrambled Eggs ➤ Appendix B	Kung Pao Chicken ➤ Chapter 6

Meal Plan Week 2: Small Meals—continued

	Snack 2	Dinner	Snack 3
Monday	Fruit and Cheese Kebabs ➤ Chapter 9 2 ounces beef jerky	Instant Pot® Salmon with Lemon and Dill ➤ Chapter 7	Black Bean Brownies ➤ Chapter 10
Tuesday	Air-Fried Tofu ➤ Chapter 8 Sweet and Sour Sauce ➤ Chapter 9	Instant Pot® Salmon with Lemon and Dill ➤ Chapter 7	Black Bean Brownies ➤ Chapter 10
Wednesday	Fruit and Cheese Kebabs ➤ Chapter 9 2 ounces beef jerky	Basil, Eggplant, and Tofu Stir-Fry ➤ Chapter 8	Black Bean Brownies ➤ Chapter 10
Thursday	Air-Fried Tofu ➤ Chapter 8 Sweet and Sour Sauce ➤ Chapter 9	Basil, Eggplant, and Tofu Stir-Fry ➤ Chapter 8	Black Bean Brownies ➤ Chapter 10
Friday	Spaghetti Squash Pizza Bites ➤ Chapter 9	Slow Cooker Chicken Cacciatore ➤ Chapter 6	Black Bean Brownies ➤ Chapter 10
Saturday	Spaghetti Squash Pizza Bites ➤ Chapter 9	Slow Cooker Chicken Cacciatore ➤ Chapter 6	Black Bean Brownies ➤ Chapter 10
Sunday	Spaghetti Squash Pizza Bites ➤ Chapter 9	Slow Cooker Chicken Cacciatore ➤ Chapter 6	Black Bean Brownies ➤ Chapter 10

As you wean off GLP-1, you'll need to gradually increase your caloric intake. This meal plan boosts your calories to help your body adjust.

	Breakfast	Lunch
Meal Plan Week 1: Transition		
Monday	Ham and Egg Cups ► Chapter 9 Simple Chocolate Protein Shake ► Appendix B	Egg-Cellent Salad ► Chapter 8 2 slices whole-grain sandwich bread
Tuesday	Ham and Egg Cups ► Chapter 9 Simple Chocolate Protein Shake ► Appendix B	Egg-Cellent Salad ► Chapter 8 2 slices whole-grain sandwich bread
Wednesday	Ham and Egg Cups ► Chapter 9 Simple Chocolate Protein Shake ► Appendix B	Egg-Cellent Salad ► Chapter 8 2 slices whole-grain sandwich bread
Thursday	Overnight Maple Walnut N'Oatmeal ► Chapter 5 Simple Vanilla Protein Shake ► Appendix B	Egg-Cellent Salad ► Chapter 8 2 slices whole-grain sandwich bread
Friday	Overnight Maple Walnut N'Oatmeal ► Chapter 5 Simple Vanilla Protein Shake ► Appendix B	Slow Cooker Chicken Chili Verde ► Chapter 6 3/4 cup brown rice
Saturday	Chili Masala Tofu Scramble ► Chapter 5 Simple Vanilla Protein Shake ► Appendix B	Lemon Tempeh with Zucchini Pasta in Sweet Honey Yogurt ► Chapter 8
Sunday	Chili Masala Tofu Scramble ► Chapter 5 Simple Vanilla Protein Shake ► Appendix B	Lemon Tempeh with Zucchini Pasta in Sweet Honey Yogurt ► Chapter 8

Meal Plan Week 1: Transition—continued

	Snack	Dinner
Monday	1 cup low-fat cottage cheese and $1/2$ cup raspberries	Slow Cooker Chicken Chili Verde ► Chapter 6 $3/4$ cup brown rice
Tuesday	1 cup low-fat cottage cheese and $1/2$ cup raspberries	Slow Cooker Chicken Chili Verde ► Chapter 6 $3/4$ cup brown rice
Wednesday	1 cup low-fat cottage cheese and $1/2$ cup raspberries	Slow Cooker Chicken Chili Verde ► Chapter 6 $3/4$ cup brown rice
Thursday	Air-Fried Crispy Chickpeas ► Chapter 9	Chicken and Bean Tacos ► Chapter 6
Friday	Air-Fried Crispy Chickpeas ► Chapter 9	Chicken and Bean Tacos ► Chapter 6
Saturday	Air-Fried Crispy Chickpeas ► Chapter 9	Chicken and Bean Tacos ► Chapter 6
Sunday	Air-Fried Crispy Chickpeas ► Chapter 9	Chicken and Bean Tacos ► Chapter 6

Meal Plan Week 2: Transition		
	Breakfast	**Lunch**
Monday	Tempeh, Tomato, and Spinach Omelet ➤ Chapter 5 Chocolate Peanut Butter Smoothie ➤ Chapter 5	Slow Cooker Chicken and Vegetable Soup ➤ Chapter 6
Tuesday	Tempeh, Tomato, and Spinach Omelet ➤ Chapter 5 Chocolate Peanut Butter Smoothie ➤ Chapter 5	Slow Cooker Chicken and Vegetable Soup ➤ Chapter 6
Wednesday	Tempeh, Tomato, and Spinach Omelet ➤ Chapter 5 Chocolate Peanut Butter Smoothie ➤ Chapter 5	Slow Cooker Chicken and Vegetable Soup ➤ Chapter 6
Thursday	Tempeh, Tomato, and Spinach Omelet ➤ Chapter 5 Chocolate Peanut Butter Smoothie ➤ Chapter 5	Slow Cooker Chicken and Vegetable Soup ➤ Chapter 6
Friday	Chicken and Vegetable Frittata ➤ Chapter 6 Chocolate Peanut Butter Smoothie ➤ Chapter 5	Chicken, Rice, and Broccoli ➤ Appendix B
Saturday	Chicken and Vegetable Frittata ➤ Chapter 6 Cinnamon Smoothie ➤ Chapter 5	Chicken, Rice, and Broccoli ➤ Appendix B
Sunday	Chicken and Vegetable Frittata ➤ Chapter 6 Cinnamon Smoothie ➤ Chapter 5	Chicken, Rice, and Broccoli ➤ Appendix B

Meal Plan Week 2: Transition—continued

	Snack	Dinner
Monday	1/2 cup plain low-fat Greek yogurt and 1/4 cup blueberries	Pot Roast with Root Vegetables ➤ Chapter 6
Tuesday	1/2 serving Pepperoni Cheese Bites ➤ Chapter 9	Pot Roast with Root Vegetables ➤ Chapter 6
Wednesday	1/2 cup plain low-fat Greek yogurt and 1/4 cup blueberries	Pot Roast with Root Vegetables ➤ Chapter 6
Thursday	1/2 serving Pepperoni Cheese Bites ➤ Chapter 9	Pot Roast with Root Vegetables ➤ Chapter 6
Friday	1/2 cup plain low-fat Greek yogurt and 1/4 cup blueberries	Tangy Sirloin Salad ➤ Chapter 6
Saturday	1/2 serving Pepperoni Cheese Bites ➤ Chapter 9	Tangy Sirloin Salad ➤ Chapter 6
Sunday	1/2 cup plain low-fat Greek yogurt and 1/4 cup blueberries	Tangy Sirloin Salad ➤ Chapter 6

Additional Recipes

Soft Scrambled Eggs on Toast

SERVES 3	
Calories	277
Fat	10g
Sodium	383mg
Carbohydrates	25g
Fiber	1g
Sugar	0g
Protein	17g

3/4 teaspoon unsalted butter

6 large eggs, beaten

3 (1.75-ounce) slices sourdough bread, toasted

1½ tablespoons chopped chives

1 Melt butter in a medium skillet over medium-low heat.
2 Add eggs to the pan and move them around with a spatula continuously. Keep pushing eggs around the skillet until fluffy and barely set, about 2 minutes.
3 Spoon eggs onto toast and sprinkle with chives. Serve immediately.

Simple Vanilla Protein Shake

SERVES 1	
Calories	210
Fat	4.5g
Sodium	140mg
Carbohydrates	2g
Fiber	1g
Sugar	0g
Protein	20g

2/3 cup Fairlife 2% Reduced Fat Ultra-Filtered Milk

1/4 cup vanilla protein powder

6 large ice cubes

Combine all ingredients in a blender and blend until thick and creamy. Serve immediately.

Oil-Free Scrambled Egg Whites

1 cup egg whites

Place egg whites in a small cold saucepan. Place over medium-low heat and stir continuously with a heat-safe spatula until fluffy and cooked through, about 10 minutes. Serve hot.

SERVES 1	
Calories	126
Fat	0g
Sodium	403mg
Carbohydrates	2g
Fiber	0g
Sugar	2g
Protein	26g

Simple Chocolate Protein Shake

$2/3$ cup Fairlife 2% Reduced Fat Ultra-Filtered Milk
$1/4$ cup chocolate protein powder
6 large ice cubes

Combine all ingredients in a blender and blend until thick and creamy. Serve immediately.

SERVES 1	
Calories	210
Fat	4.5g
Sodium	140mg
Carbohydrates	2g
Fiber	1g
Sugar	0g
Protein	20g

Scrambled Eggs

SERVES 1	
Calories	210
Fat	12g
Sodium	293mg
Carbohydrates	1g
Fiber	0g
Sugar	1g
Protein	22g

$^1/_2$ teaspoon olive oil

2 large eggs, beaten

2 large egg whites, beaten (approximately $^1/_3$ cup)

1 Heat oil in a medium skillet over medium heat.

2 Add eggs and egg whites to the pan and move them around with a spatula continuously. Keep pushing mixture around the skillet until fluffy and barely set, about 2 minutes. Serve immediately.

Chicken, Rice, and Broccoli

2 cups water

1 cup brown rice

1 pound boneless, skinless chicken breast

2 tablespoons olive oil

1/2 teaspoon salt

4 cups chopped broccoli

SERVES 4	
Calories	396
Fat	12g
Sodium	381mg
Carbohydrates	41g
Fiber	4g
Sugar	2g
Protein	31g

1 Preheat oven to 400°F. Line a small baking dish with parchment paper.

2 Place water in a medium saucepan and bring to a boil over high heat. Stir in rice, cover, and reduce heat to medium-low. Simmer for 40 minutes or until water is absorbed. Fluff rice with a fork.

3 Brush chicken with oil and sprinkle with salt. Place in the prepared baking dish. Bake for 25–30 minutes until cooked through. Cool slightly, then cut into slices.

4 In a large pot with a steaming basket, bring 1" water to a boil. Add broccoli to the steaming basket, cover, and steam for 5 minutes or until tender.

5 Divide rice, chicken, and broccoli among four plates or storage containers. Serve immediately or refrigerate for up to five days.

GLP-1 Food Lists

Foods to Eat While Taking GLP-1 Medications

LEAN PROTEINS

- Beef, lean cuts (in moderation)
- Chicken
- Eggs
- Fish
- Tofu and tempeh
- Turkey

WHOLE GRAINS

- Barley
- Brown rice
- Bulgur
- Farro
- Millet
- Oats
- Popcorn
- Quinoa
- Whole wheat
- Wild rice

NON-STARCHY VEGETABLES AND FRUITS

- Apples
- Avocados
- Beets
- Bell peppers
- Berries
- Cantaloupe
- Carrots
- Celery
- Collard greens
- Cucumbers
- Eggplant
- Ginger
- Grapefruit
- Jicama
- Kale
- Kiwis
- Leafy greens
- Lemons
- Lettuce
- Mushrooms
- Oranges
- Peaches
- Spinach
- Squash
- Tomatoes
- Watermelon

BEANS AND LEGUMES

- ○ Black beans
- ○ Chickpeas
- ○ Edamame
- ○ Kidney beans
- ○ Lentils
- ○ Pinto beans
- ○ White beans

NUTS AND SEEDS

- ○ Almonds
- ○ Cashews
- ○ Chia seeds
- ○ Flaxseeds
- ○ Nut butters
- ○ Peanuts
- ○ Pistachios
- ○ Pumpkin seeds
- ○ Walnuts

DAIRY PRODUCTS

- ○ Cottage cheese
- ○ Greek yogurt
- ○ Kefir
- ○ Low-fat milk
- ○ Protein drinks

LOW–GLYCEMIC INDEX BEVERAGES

- ○ Black tea
- ○ Broth
- ○ Ginger tea
- ○ Green tea
- ○ Water

Foods to Avoid While Taking GLP-1 Medications

- Fried foods
- Foods high in saturated and trans fats (pizza, doughnuts, burgers, fries)
- Ultra-processed foods (chips, deli products)
- Refined carbohydrates (white bread, crackers, white flour, white rice)
- Spicy foods (hot sauce, salsa, hot peppers)
- Fatty cuts of meat (ribs, ground beef, marbled steak, pork shoulder)
- Vegetables that may cause GI upset, like asparagus, Brussels sprouts, onions, broccoli, cauliflower, cabbage (okay in moderation)
- Foods high in refined sugars (baked goods, candy, ice cream)
- High–glycemic index foods, like potatoes, cereals, pretzels, dried fruits, mangoes, pineapple (okay in moderation)
- Carbonated drinks (sodas, seltzers)
- Beverages with added sugars (juices, teas, energy drinks)
- Alcohol
- Caffeine

Tips for Success

Take "Before" Photos.

The scale doesn't show everything! Pictures are one of the best ways to track your progress over time and stay motivated.

Pay Attention to Your Carbohydrate Intake.

Carbohydrates break down into glucose when digested, and an overload of glucose can lead to weight gain. Opting for whole-grain, low-carb, or low-glycemic options can help maintain weight and provide some extra fiber as well.

Take a Walk after Meals.

Taking a walk after eating can help alleviate symptoms of delayed gastric emptying. Walking also supports better blood sugar management by preventing significant spikes after meals.

Stay Hydrated.

Drink more water than you think you need! Not only does hydration support a healthy metabolism, but dehydration can exacerbate the side effects from the medication. Feel free to add flavoring to make your water more appetizing.

Prioritize Protein.

You should aim to incorporate protein at every eating opportunity. Keep premade protein shakes on hand for days when you are struggling to reach your protein goals.

Eat Slowly.

Taking your time while eating can help you better recognize your fullness cues. Aim to stop eating when you feel about 80 percent full. The smallest amount of overeating can trigger unwanted side effects.

Make a List.

Whether or not you're tracking your intake, it can be helpful to keep a list of foods that trigger your side effects. From the start, avoid well-known culprits like high-fat foods and added sugars. As you progress, if you notice that a particular dish or product causes nausea, gastrointestinal upset, or any other side effect, make a note of it.

Advocate for Yourself.

If you are having issues with the medication, don't be afraid to speak up to your healthcare provider. There are many options for dosing and different types of medication. If you don't feel heard or seen by your provider, there are many others out there to choose from.

Additional Resources

Articles

"FDA Approves New Drug Treatment for Chronic Weight Management, First Since 2014" by the FDA

https://fda.gov/news-events/press-announcements/fda-approves-new-drug-treatment-chronic-weight-management-first-2014

Announcement of the approval of the semaglutide drug Wegovy for chronic weight management in adults with obesity or overweight with at least one weight-related condition.

"Ozempic for Weight Loss: Does It Work, and What Do Experts Recommend?" by UC Davis Health

https://health.ucdavis.edu/blog/cultivating-health/ozempic-for-weight-loss-does-it-work-and-what-do-experts-recommend/2023/07

Answers to questions about what Ozempic is and how it works.

"The Pros, Cons, and Unknowns of Popular Weight-Loss Drugs" by Emily Gaines Buchler, John Hopkins University

https://hub.jhu.edu/2024/01/11/ozempic-wegovy-weight-loss-drugs-pros-cons/

Summary of an episode of the podcast *Public Health on Call* about the safety and effectiveness of Ozempic and Wegovy, featuring two Johns Hopkins University experts.

"Semaglutide for Weight Loss—What You Need to Know" by UCLA Health

https://uclahealth.org/news/article/semaglutide-weight-loss-what-you-need-know

General information about semaglutide and who it is suitable for.

"We Know Where New Weight Loss Drugs Came From, But Not Why They Work" by Gina Kolata, *The New York Times*, August 17, 2023

https://nytimes.com/2023/08/17/health/weight-loss-drugs-obesity-ozempic-wegovy.html

Describes the origins of GLP-1 medications.

"Wegovy vs. Ozempic: The Truth about New 'Weight-Loss' Drugs" by UC Health

https://uchealth.org/today/wegovy-vs-ozempic-the-truth-about-new-weight-loss-drugs/

Outlines things to consider before starting the weight loss drugs Wegovy and Ozempic.

Apps

Carb Manager

If you experience a reduced appetite on Ozempic and want to manage carbs more carefully, this app helps you stay on track with lower-carb meal plans.

Cronometer

This app ensures you're not only managing calories but also getting all the necessary nutrients while on Ozempic, which is critical to avoid malnutrition due to reduced appetite.

StrongLifts

Weight loss on Ozempic can sometimes lead to muscle loss, and this app helps you stay focused on building and maintaining muscle mass as part of a sustainable weight loss journey.

Books

Atomic Habits: An Easy & Proven Way to Build Good Habits & Break Bad Ones by James Clear

https://jamesclear.com/atomic-habits

A system for building good habits and reducing bad ones.

The Everything® Mediterranean Diet Book by Connie Diekman and Sam Sotiropoulos

https://simonandschuster.com/books/The-Everything-Mediterranean-Diet-Book/Connie-Diekman/Everything/9781440506741

Covers the science behind healthy eating and includes 100 recipes.

The Everything® Healthy Mediterranean Cookbook by Peter Minaki

https://simonandschuster.com/books/The-Everything-Healthy-Mediterranean-Cookbook/Peter-Minaki/Everything/9781507211519

Includes 300 easy, healthy, and delicious Mediterranean recipes—many ready in 30 minutes or less.

How to Change: The Science of Getting from Where You Are to Where You Want to Be by Katy Milkman

https://katymilkman.com/book

A step-by-step guide to creating a unique plan for overcoming barriers to change.

Magic Pill: The Extraordinary Benefits and Disturbing Risks of the New Weight-Loss Drugs by Johann Hari

https://penguinrandomhouse.com/books/743989/magic-pill-by-johann-hari/

A look at the transformative new weight loss drugs and how they are changing society's relationship with food, weight, and bodies.

Mindful Eating: A Guide to Rediscovering a Healthy and Joyful Relationship with Food by Jan Chozen Bays

https://shambhala.com/mindful-eating-15034.html?srsltid=AfmBOorVX fFXU9oz_Er6M6tWnVl_lvTDDQw9QtX UbfsRWf_9BuQ307uX

A guide to changing your relationship with food.

Podcasts

Eat Move Think, "All About Semaglutide, Ozempic, Wegovy & Rybelsus"

https://eatmovethinkpodcast.com/podcast/ep180-semaglutide-ozempic-wegovy-rybelsus

The External Medicine Podcast, "Stephan Guyenet, PhD: GLP-1, Semaglutide, and the Big Future of Weight Loss Therapies"

https://podcasts.apple.com/us/podcast/stephan-guyenet-phd-glp-1-semaglutide-and-the-big/id1554007057?i=1000546823625

The Journal., "Trillion Dollar Shot, Episode 1: Birth of a Blockbuster"

https://open.spotify.com/episode/1XIgBAKpL9IEcd20MwPLKI?si=I2qUTzudQkeS7Rtf0VIuvA&nd=1&dlsi=dbe32f905c68407c

The Leading Voices in Food, "Highly Successful Weight Loss Drug Semaglutide Explained"

https://podcasts.apple.com/us/podcast/highly-successful-weight-loss-drug-semaglutide-explained/id1444757309?i=1000559472080

Studies

"Clinical Insight on Semaglutide for Chronic Weight Management in Adults: Patient Selection and Special Considerations" by Chao, et al.

https://ncbi.nlm.nih.gov/pmc/articles/PMC9807016/

"Efficacy and Safety of Semaglutide for Weight Management: Evidence from the STEP Program" by Amaro, et al.

https://tandfonline.com/doi/full/10.1080/00325481.2022.2147326

"Efficacy and Safety of Semaglutide on Weight Loss in Obese or Overweight Patients Without Diabetes: A Systematic Review and Meta-Analysis of Randomized Controlled Trials" by Gao, et al.

https://frontiersin.org/journals/pharmacology/articles/10.3389/fphar.2022.935823/full

"Long-Term Efficacy and Safety of Once-Weekly Semaglutide for Weight Loss in Patients Without Diabetes: A Systematic Review and Meta-Analysis of Randomized Controlled Trials" by Moiz, et al.

https://ajconline.org/article/S0002-9149(24)00319-9/fulltext

"Once-Weekly Semaglutide in Adults with Overweight or Obesity" by Wilding, et al.

https://nejm.org/doi/full/10.1056/NEJMoa2032183

"Oral Semaglutide 50 mg Taken Once per Day in Adults with Overweight or Obesity (OASIS 1): A Randomised, Double-Blind, Placebo-Controlled, Phase 3 Trial" by Knop, et al.

https://thelancet.com/journals/lancet/article/PIIS0140-6736(23)01185-6/abstract

"Wegovy (Semaglutide): A New Weight Loss Drug for Chronic Weight Management" by Singh, et al.

https://journals.sagepub.com/doi/10.1136/jim-2021-001952

"Weight Loss Outcomes Associated with Semaglutide Treatment for Patients with Overweight or Obesity" by Ghusn, et al.

https://ncbi.nlm.nih.gov/pmc/articles/PMC9486455/

STANDARD US/METRIC MEASUREMENT CONVERSIONS

VOLUME CONVERSIONS

US Volume Measure	Metric Equivalent
⅛ teaspoon	0.5 milliliter
¼ teaspoon	1 milliliter
½ teaspoon	2 milliliters
1 teaspoon	5 milliliters
½ tablespoon	7 milliliters
1 tablespoon (3 teaspoons)	15 milliliters
2 tablespoons (1 fluid ounce)	30 milliliters
¼ cup (4 tablespoons)	60 milliliters
⅓ cup	90 milliliters
½ cup (4 fluid ounces)	125 milliliters
⅔ cup	160 milliliters
¾ cup (6 fluid ounces)	180 milliliters
1 cup (16 tablespoons)	250 milliliters
1 pint (2 cups)	500 milliliters
1 quart (4 cups)	1 liter (about)

WEIGHT CONVERSIONS

US Weight Measure	Metric Equivalent
½ ounce	15 grams
1 ounce	30 grams
2 ounces	60 grams
3 ounces	85 grams
¼ pound (4 ounces)	115 grams
½ pound (8 ounces)	225 grams
¾ pound (12 ounces)	340 grams
1 pound (16 ounces)	454 grams

OVEN TEMPERATURE CONVERSIONS

Degrees Fahrenheit	Degrees Celsius
200 degrees F	95 degrees C
250 degrees F	120 degrees C
275 degrees F	135 degrees C
300 degrees F	150 degrees C
325 degrees F	160 degrees C
350 degrees F	180 degrees C
375 degrees F	190 degrees C
400 degrees F	205 degrees C
425 degrees F	220 degrees C
450 degrees F	230 degrees C

BAKING PAN SIZES

American	Metric
8 × 1½ inch round baking pan	20 × 4 cm cake tin
9 × 1½ inch round baking pan	23 × 3.5 cm cake tin
11 × 7 × 1½ inch baking pan	28 × 18 × 4 cm baking tin
13 × 9 × 2 inch baking pan	30 × 20 × 5 cm baking tin
2 quart rectangular baking dish	30 × 20 × 3 cm baking tin
15 × 10 × 2 inch baking pan	30 × 25 × 2 cm baking tin (Swiss roll tin)
9 inch pie plate	22 × 4 or 23 × 4 cm pie plate
7 or 8 inch springform pan	18 or 20 cm springform or loose bottom cake tin
9 × 5 × 3 inch loaf pan	23 × 13 × 7 cm or 2 lb narrow loaf or pate tin
1½ quart casserole	1.5 liter casserole
2 quart casserole	2 liter casserole

Index

Adapted Material List